MANUAL FOR THE RECOVERY ROOM

MANUAL FOR THE RECOVERY ROOM

Stanton Belinkoff, M.D.
Director, Department of Anesthesia
St. Luke's Hospital
New Bedford, Massachusetts

FOREWORD by Philip S. Marcus, M.D.
Director, Department of Anesthesia
Boston City Hospital, Boston

LITTLE, BROWN AND COMPANY
Boston

Copyright © 1967 by Little, Brown and Company (Inc.)

All rights reserved. No part of this book may be reproduced in any form without written permission from the publisher.

Library of Congress catalog card No. 66-29833

First Edition

Published in Great Britain
by J. & A. Churchill Ltd., London

Printed in the United States of America

To
MILLICENT

FOREWORD

DURING THE PAST TWO DECADES the recovery room has become an integral part of most modern hospitals. It forms a vital link between the operating room and the patient's return to the haven of his hospital bed. Because of the physiological effects of anesthesia and surgery, the patient must be observed and cared for by a highly trained, specialized group of personnel before he can be safely returned to an area of less-intensive care.

The knowledge and skills required in a properly functioning recovery room are not usually attained in any one place or at any one time during the educational process of the physician or the nurse. Manual for the Recovery Room could have been written only by someone who has had continuous and intimate contact with the daily professional and organizational problems of this highly specialized unit. The anesthesiologist is usually the supervisor of such units and as such is best qualified to describe its function. Dr. Belinkoff has written in simple terminology a highly practical and clinically applicable manual for the use and training of all personnel who become part of this essential division of the modern hospital. In my opinion he has rendered a great service to all who wish to establish such a unit or who, having once created a recovery room, desire to keep at hand a set of guidelines and pertinent information for its most efficient functioning.

PHILIP S. MARCUS

PREFACE

THE CONCEPT of the recovery room is a major advance in patient care that has achieved wide acceptance in the last twenty years. In most hospitals it has become an indispensable part of the postoperative surgical and anesthetic care of the patient. Its obvious advantages have made the recovery room essential to any hospital with an active surgical service. So far as is known, no hospital has discontinued the use of its recovery room.

When recovery rooms were originally established, patients were held for periods ranging from an hour to several days. However, with the growth in intensive care units in recent years, the recovery room should now be regarded more as a postanesthesia room. The patient should thus be kept only until he has recovered from the anesthesia and its effects. When he becomes a surgical problem without superimposed anesthesia effects, he should be transferred either to a surgical unit or to an intensive care unit, depending upon the circumstances and routine of the hospital.

This book is an outgrowth of a series of classes, lectures, and demonstrations held for the recovery room personnel at St. Luke's Hospital, New Bedford, Massachusetts. The many questions and interest expressed pointed up the need for a manual that would explain the basic concepts involved, their relation to the problems in this particular period of the patient's stay, and the means of improving patient care in this area. Anatomy and physiology are covered in brief and rudimentary fashion to explain the respiratory and circulatory systems.

This presentation, therefore, attempts to explain and clarify the status, management, and function of the recovery room and to support the opinions expressed herein.

S. B.

New Bedford, Massachusetts

CONTENTS

FOREWORD by Philip S. Marcus	vii
PREFACE	ix

1. GENERAL CONSIDERATIONS — 1
The Need for a Recovery Room	2
Training Recovery Room Personnel	3

2. ORGANIZATION, ADMINISTRATION, AND PERSONNEL — 5
The Role of the Anesthesiologist	5
The Role of the Nurse	6
The Role of the Supervisor	7
Personnel Policies	9
Recovery Room Management	10
The Role of the Physician	13
Discharging the Patient	14
Financial Considerations	14

3. PHYSICAL AND ARCHITECTURAL CONSIDERATIONS — 17
Room Arrangement	18

Heat Regulation 24
Oxygen and Suction 25
Nurse's Station 26

4. EQUIPMENT 29
Drug Supply 31
Miscellaneous Equipment 32
Electronic Equipment 33

5. RESPIRATION 35
Anatomy and Organs of Respiration 35
Mechanics of Respiration 39
Regulation of Respiration 41
Practical Considerations 43
Respiratory Obstruction 47
Respiration and Ventilation 51

6. CIRCULATION 59
Anatomy and Physiology 59
Practical Considerations 63
Shock 66

7. EMERGENCE FROM ANESTHESIA 75
Cyclopropane 76

Ether	77
Halothane	77
Ethyl Chloride	78
Nitrous Oxide	78
Narcotic Anesthesia	79
Intravenous Barbiturates	79
Rectal Anesthesia	80
Spinal Anesthesia	81
Relaxants	83

8. PATIENT CARE — 85
   - Stir-up Regime — 86
   - Blood Transfusion Reactions — 88
   - Hypertension in the Immediate Postoperative Period — 90
   - Hypotension in the Immediate Postoperative Period — 91
   - Control and Prevention of Infection — 92

9. SPECIALIZED PROCEDURES — 95
   - Care of the Patient Following Thoracotomy — 95
   - Care of the Pediatric Patient — 100
   - Care of the Neurosurgical Patient—Specifically Following Intracranial Surgery — 103
   - Care of the Orthopedic Patient — 105
   - Care of the Urological Patient — 106

xiv / Contents

10. CARDIAC ARREST 109
　　Sudden Collapse or Arrest 109
　　Diagnosis 110
　　Treatment 111

APPENDIX 115

SUGGESTED SUPPLEMENTAL
　　READING 121

INDEX 123

MANUAL FOR THE RECOVERY ROOM

1
GENERAL CONSIDERATIONS

THE RECOVERY ROOM is, specifically, an area to which patients are brought following an operative procedure to recover from the effects of the anesthetic. They are watched and cared for by specialized personnel until such time as they are fully conscious and able to return to the ward without danger of such immediate postanesthetic complications as asphyxia, shock, and respiratory or circulatory collapse. If the patient has had major surgery or has other problems of a medical nature not associated with the anesthesia, he should go to an intensive care unit or to a ward with special nursing attention.

The recovery room should be carefully differentiated from a postoperative or general intensive care unit. The recovery room is, in reality, a postanesthesia room. A postsurgical room is an area where the patient may be retained for periods of several days or more until he has recovered from the effects of the surgery. An intensive care unit may keep both medical and surgical patients for varying and indefinite periods of time for specialized care and close observation. These various aspects of patient care may all be conducted in one area or in different areas of the hospital. For the purposes of this discussion, the recovery room will be considered only as a postanesthesia room. This is true in our hospital and, I think, in most active general hospitals of medium size.

THE NEED FOR A RECOVERY ROOM

There are a number of advantages to having a recovery room: (1) The room permits centralization and grouping of the patients requiring this kind of care. (2) Equipment and personnel are all specialized. (3) The facilities, which are also specialized, can be provided in one place rather than scattered throughout the hospital. The recovery room can save lives and also decrease the hospital stay of the patient by providing the best possible care during this critical postsurgical period. This is true regardless of the nature of the hospital—voluntary, military, or city—and irrespective of whether the patient is going to a private or semiprivate room or a ward. The acute shortage of trained nursing personnel, which probably will not be alleviated in the foreseeable future, makes specialized areas of this type very important, especially in view of the shortage of special duty nurses. Since nursing personnel on the wards are busy and inadequate in numbers, much patient care must be left in the hands of aides and assistants of varying degrees of training and experience. In general, since postoperative patients require more than ordinary nursing care, it is essential that they be placed in an area that is adjusted to their requirements.

All general, or even specialized, hospitals that do any significant amount of surgery should have a specific area such as a recovery room to which patients go upon leaving the operating room. This recovery room should be located as close as possible to the operating room so that surgeons and anesthesiologists can be available in case of emergency. In our hospital we consider the recovery room as an extension of the operating room. It is in the operating room suite, and the personnel are under the administrative control of the operating room supervisor and under the medical control of the anesthesia department.

TRAINING RECOVERY ROOM PERSONNEL

All patients should go to the recovery room regardless of whether they have had spinal, some form of regional, or a general anesthetic; all may present problems in the immediate postoperative period. Nursing personnel should be aware of these problems and be trained in the use of such special apparatus as suction machines and respiratory assistance equipment. They should be trained in intravenous therapy, or at least in the performance of venipuncture, so that solutions can be restarted or administered when ordered without calling a physician.

The period when patients are awakening from an anesthetic is really a stage intermediate between the immediate supervision of the anesthesiologist during the operative procedure and the time when they will be placed on general care on the surgical ward. In order to maintain a high standard of care, the supervising nurse should have had special training and have been made aware of the physiological problems that may arise, especially in the patient who has been asleep during an operative procedure and is now regaining his sensorium.

The problems of respiratory physiology, circulatory dynamics, their basic physiology, causes of trouble, and definitive measures of treatment that can be taken should all be considered in the training of personnel in the recovery room. They should be able to care for minor emergencies but, at the same time, have available capable physicians who will respond quickly to help with problems that they feel are beyond their own capacities. Training of all personnel in the recovery room should encompass: (1) prevention of respiratory obstruction; (2) generalized care of the patient; (3) a knowledge of the immediate postoperative problems that may arise in respect to specialized types of surgery; and (4) emergency treatment of circulatory catastrophes.

2
ORGANIZATION, ADMINISTRATION, AND PERSONNEL

THE ROLE OF THE ANESTHESIOLOGIST

The recovery room should be under the immediate supervision, and be the responsibility, of the anesthesia department. From a medical point of view, the anesthesiologists are readily available, are in the hospital most or all of the day, and are the only physicians constantly in the operating room. Many surgeons work in the operating room; they come, do their cases, and then leave. They go to their offices, make rounds, go out on calls, or are otherwise immediately unavailable for the myriad problems that may arise in caring for the patient. It has therefore been considered advisable in most institutions to make the anesthesia department along with the surgeon directly responsible for the care of the patient in the recovery room.

Problems of respiration and of circulation can usually be handled by the anesthesiologists, who are best equipped to do so by reason of their specialized knowledge of physiology and pharmacology, in addition to general medical training and wide experience in observing the direct and immediate actions of drugs. Other problems that may arise relative to the surgery performed may be handled by either the anesthesiologist, the surgeon, or both. We feel that minor problems that do not require major surgical judgment or intervention can be taken care of in the normal course of events. However, we do not hesitate to contact the surgeon, who responds immediately and dramatically, if there is any question in our minds about the patient's condition or about complications for which there seem to be no obvious reasons. It is noteworthy that the surgical department generally is happy to delegate its problems during this period and usually offers excellent cooperation.

THE ROLE OF THE NURSE

The second half of the team caring for the patient in the recovery room is the nursing department. Here we come into what may be a gray area in that the nurses should be directly responsible to the anesthesiologists and to their orders. Some of the rules and regulations for the nurse in other areas of the hospital should not apply; dependence on general nursing authority must be eliminated to facilitate immediate decisions and quick and efficient care.

The recovery room may be set up under the overall supervision of the operating room supervisor, or may be a separate unit, depending on both the physical layout and the personnel of each individual institution. If the recovery room is an integral part of the operating room and actually in the operating room suite, then it would seem advisable for the operating room supervisor to control the staffs of both the recovery room and the operating room. This would be the ideal situation since all nonmedical, or at least non-physician, personnel in the entire area would be under one supervisor. Interchange of personnel and auxiliary help such as orderlies and aides, to make the most efficient use of their efforts, would be much easier. If, however, space is not available in the immediate operating room area and the recovery room is any distance from it, even though on the same floor, then the recovery room should be set up as a totally independent unit with its own supervisor and auxiliary personnel. In either case, even if the recovery room is a subdivision of the operating room, there should still be a graduate nurse, specially trained in the care of these patients, in immediate charge.

THE ROLE OF THE SUPERVISOR

The choice of a head nurse in this area is extremely important. While she and the entire department will inevitably be part of the nursing service, their position is different from that of the nurses in the other wards in the hospital since they are immediately responsible to the anesthesia department. When setting up an organization and recruiting personnel, individual effort and attention must be given to the head nurse to see that she is offered specialized training and that she profits by it. The fact that a nurse has proved very adequate on the average ward does not mean that she will be able to carry out the duties required in the recovery room as well as she could perform administrative work on the average surgical or medical floor. The recovery room nurse must be adept at both recognizing and starting the treatment of respiratory and circulatory emergencies. Also, in emergencies she must not feel so proficient that she makes no effort to obtain help from available physicians. It is not easy to acquire such a person, but she is essential to the proper and most efficient operation of an area of this nature.

The recovery room supervisor must be interested in this type of work and should have had a good generalized basis in nursing, both surgical and medical. She should have had some experience as an operating room nurse to give her some understanding of the trauma the patient has already undergone in order to better understand his condition when he arrives in the recovery room. A continuing series of lectures and practical demonstrations by the anesthesia department and talks by the various surgical specialists should be given to the entire recovery room staff to make them aware of the individual needs of the different surgeons and their patients.

Student nurses of any grade, whether from a nursing school or a practical nursing school, when rotated through the recovery room should serve only as observers and should not be allowed to undertake any large measure of patient care. They should not be given any responsibility and should be under constant supervision even during simple patient contacts.

PERSONNEL POLICIES

The number of personnel required should be determined after a study of such factors as the size of the hospital, the number of operative procedures done during the day, the anesthetics most commonly used, and the patient flow. In addition to a well-qualified supervisor, additional registered nurses, aides, and orderlies should be employed in numbers sufficient to assure adequate patient care and attention. This recovery, or postanesthesia, room should generally be staffed so as to remain open as long as required to care for the patients on the average operating schedule. Considering ourselves an average institution, with a predominantly morning operating schedule that progressively decreases until 3:00 P.M. each day, we have found that two shifts are adequate. The bulk of the personnel are here on a staggered basis from 7:00 in the morning until 5:00 in the afternoon. Our schedule starts at 7:30, and patients begin to arrive in the recovery room by 8:00 A.M. Our personnel come at different hours; first at 7:00, next at 8:00, and the majority at 8:30 A.M. Our maximum patient load is during the hours of 10:00 to 1:00; then, as the patient census falls, our personnel start leaving. Thus, our attendants leave between 3:00 and 4:30 P.M. During the period from 4:30 to 11:00 at night, only one nurse is available, since all the normally scheduled cases have been returned to their rooms by 4:30 or 5:00. Patients who remain may have had a very long and difficult procedure and require extra care. We also have the normal emergent patient operative procedures, which are scheduled for from about 4:30 to 6:00 P.M., a period corresponding with the close of office hours for the average surgeon.

RECOVERY ROOM MANAGEMENT

Individual considerations may be taken into account in determining the number of beds required in the recovery room. The average nursing division is depleted of some of its personnel during the lunch hour; to ease their burden, we have established a policy of not returning patients to their wards between 11:30 and 1:00 o'clock, even though they have fully recovered from the anesthetic and are wide-awake. Although it has increased our space requirements somewhat and has created a tendency to temporary overcrowding, we feel that the patients receive much better care during this period by being kept in the recovery room rather than being sent to different wards that are critically short of personnel during the lunch hour.

Ideally, a nurse anesthetist is assigned to remain in the recovery room if others are available in the anesthesia department. This procedure provides a person extremely well trained in respiratory problems, since a nurse anesthetist is trained and experienced in managing airways and performing the respiratory resuscitative measures that are the immediate and most frequent problems in the recovery room. However, since such nurses are in short supply and command much higher compensation than the average registered nurse, it is sometimes impractical to employ them for this purpose. Moreover, the trained nurse anesthetist may not be willing to undertake such responsibility. However, if a school for nurse anesthetists is being conducted in a hospital, rotation of such students through the recovery room is advisable both for their training and to provide a useful addition to the personnel. Nurse's aides in the recovery room, when trained in determining such factors as blood pressure and pulse, can check the patients after they have reacted from the anesthesia and during the period when they are being watched to assure that they are stabilized. Such work is, of course, done under the supervision of the head nurse.

In general, it is not advisable for graduate nurses to rotate through the recovery room, since they must have specialized training in order to be useful here. The average graduate nurse from other sections of the hospital will find herself lost in the recovery room. This is even truer where a recovery room has been in existence for some time and the nurses on the floors have consequently lost contact with the immediate postoperative patient. Since nurses have now become accustomed to receiving their patients from the recovery room in a conscious condition, fully recovered from the anesthesia, they are no longer familiar with the many individual problems that may arise and are not capable of handling them. Therefore, it is essential to establish an independent staff of specially trained people who are able and willing to do this work. As additional personnel, operating room nurses should receive some training in the recovery room so that, if they are needed for any reason such as sickness or vacations, they may step into the breach.

A resident should be assigned to the recovery room as part of his rotation and training in those hospitals that have active teaching programs. It is an integral part of both surgical and anesthesia training to become aware of the problems of the patient emerging from anesthesia. Much can be learned here. However, in the average hospital anesthesia residents and anesthesiologists are few in number, generally making it impossible to have a physician in constant attendance; the training of the nurse in charge thus assumes even greater importance. However, this lack may be remedied and adequate supervisory care furnished if the individual anesthesiologists adopt a policy of passing through the recovery room on their way to and from the operating room to check the patients and consult with the charge nurse when they bring a patient in. It is obvious that close cooperation is essential between the nurses and other personnel in the recovery room, on the one hand and the anesthesiologists, on the other.

Since all patients must go to the recovery room, a problem may sometimes arise with private duty nurses. It is usually advisable not to permit them in the area; they are unaccustomed to the routine and unfamiliar with the techniques of care. Rather than have them in the way, we routinely require private nurses to stay in the patients' rooms and have everything in readiness for their return.

Visitors are not permitted in the recovery room at any time, with the exception of the immediate family if the patient is in extremis. In this circumstance, the patient is isolated by curtains and may be seen for a very short time by the immediate family or by the clergy if death appears imminent.

THE ROLE OF THE PHYSICIAN

Either the anesthesiologist or the anesthetist should accompany the patient to his position in the recovery room. Here he should be met by the charge nurse and should tell her anything specific or unusual that has occurred to this particular patient and warn her of anything out of the ordinary that may happen in the immediate postoperative period. The anesthesia record should be completely filled out so that the nurse can immediately know what anesthesia was given, what operative procedure was performed, and what the patient's general condition was at the close of the procedure. At the same time, the surgeon should write his postoperative orders and communicate to the nurse any facts that he feels are important. A discussion of postoperative fluids and other specific items that may be necessary for the patient during this period should not only be written down, but should be discussed orally between the surgeon or the anesthesiologist and the recovery room supervisor.

DISCHARGING THE PATIENT

Under average circumstances, the recovery room supervisor decides when a patient is to be discharged and sent to his room. This is done when, in her judgment, the patient has fully reacted from the anesthesia and will not be affected detrimentally by the transfer. In unusual cases, this decision should be made in consultation with a physician, but with experience the supervisor will be able to decide properly when the average patient should be moved. Criteria should be: (1) when the patient has regained consciousness and is oriented as to time and place; (2) when the airway is clear and danger of vomiting and aspiration is past; and (3) when his circulatory and vital signs are stabilized.

FINANCIAL CONSIDERATIONS

The philosophy of establishing charges for patient services has, in recent years, been revised in that it is now a widely accepted policy to establish each patient service area as a separate cost center and to base the patient charges accordingly.

Each patient using the recovery room facility should be billed on a charge factor that will make the recovery room a self-sustaining unit. A suggested method is to price the patient service in direct relationship to the time the patient utilizes the recovery room: for example, $7.00 to $10.00 for the first hour and $2.00 for each succeeding hour. A less equitable arrangement would involve a flat charge for the use of the recovery room. In order to establish a proper base on which to compute equitable charges, the recovery room's direct operating expenses must be identified and summarized by separate expense accounts. Indirect costs, such as those of administration and maintenance, should be allocated in conformity with generally accepted accounting principles.

Many hospitals do not separate recovery room and operating room costs. Consequently, specific charges cannot be made for the use of the recovery room area. Under this method patients are charged for the combined services of the operating and recovery areas. This may prove less than satisfactory, as the utilization of the recovery room does not always relate proportionately to the length of the operating room procedure.

Care should be exercised to develop complete costs, both direct and indirect, and to compile statistical information so that sufficient income will be realized under either charge method.

3
PHYSICAL AND ARCHITECTURAL CONSIDERATIONS

THE RECOVERY ROOM should be located as close as possible to the operating room suite, if not actually in it. The greater the proximity, the easier it becomes to give close supervision and the more readily available will be the anesthesiological or surgical aid that may be required at times. If the recovery room is any distance from the operating room or on another floor, it tends to become isolated and regarded as a disassociated, independent area and not as an intimately integrated part of the period of emergence from surgery and anesthesia. Every effort should therefore be directed to having the recovery room in, or immediately adjacent to, the operating room area.

There are basically two types of recovery rooms: (1) Those in new buildings, where they were planned as an integral part of the building. This permits taking into account all the important features to be considered as regards proximity to the operating room and physical size, which can be done in a building program when all factors can be considered and incorporated during the planning stages. (2) Those in hospitals with an existing plant that is not being changed or enlarged and recognize the need for a recovery room, but must incorporate it into finished structure, with existing walls, some of which cannot be moved. Such rooms are sometimes very makeshift; sometimes they may work out well. Obviously, those planned as new units will be more efficient and better located. The recovery room is now important enough to warrant great efforts to ensure its proper functioning. Examples of recovery room layouts are shown in Figure 1.

ROOM ARRANGEMENT

It is not necessary to have any subdivision either as to sex of patient or the type of anesthesia received. As long as normal care is taken to prevent exposure of patients, males and females can be watched simultaneously in the same recovery room. The patients are all on stretchers or beds with sides, are covered with blankets, and may be separated by curtains when necessary. The increased efficiency of care should override any imaginary overstepping of the bounds of propriety. If the recovery room is physically divided into areas, separate staffs must be present in each area to observe the patients adequately. This unnecessarily increases the staffing demands without providing better patient care. It is important that all patients be positioned so that they are readily and continually seen by the personnel and not subdivided into rooms where they may be overlooked or where an emergency is not immediately evident.

It is best that the recovery room be set up to incorporate the nurse's station. Personnel should not be required to leave the room at frequent intervals for supplies. The charting desk and supply cabinets, but not the cleanup areas, should be placed so that personnel, while attending to their chores, will still have the patients in plain view. An arrangement where the nurse's station or charting area is outside the room or isolated from it in any way is not acceptable. The desk should be so arranged that a nurse occupying it faces the patients and does not have her back to them; this is a common error. Arrangements can be made to isolate a patient, possibly for placement of a catheter or for other types of personal care. In general, however, the room should be continuously open to view, and patients should be placed so that they can all be seen immediately at a glance.

Segregation of Children

One concession may be made in segregating pediatric patients from adults; if a sufficient volume of pediatric work is being done, this is advisable. In hospitals with an active ear, nose, and throat service performing three or more tonsillectomies a day on children, a segregated area may be established for these youngsters, whose emergence from anesthesia is often distressing to adults. They must, however, still be under the immediate care of a nurse who is not required simultaneously to attend patients in the adult recovery room. In some hospitals, the surgeon may

NO WINDOWS NECESSARY

NEW RECOVERY ROOM

GRAPHIC SCALE IN FEET: 0 1 2 3 4 5 6

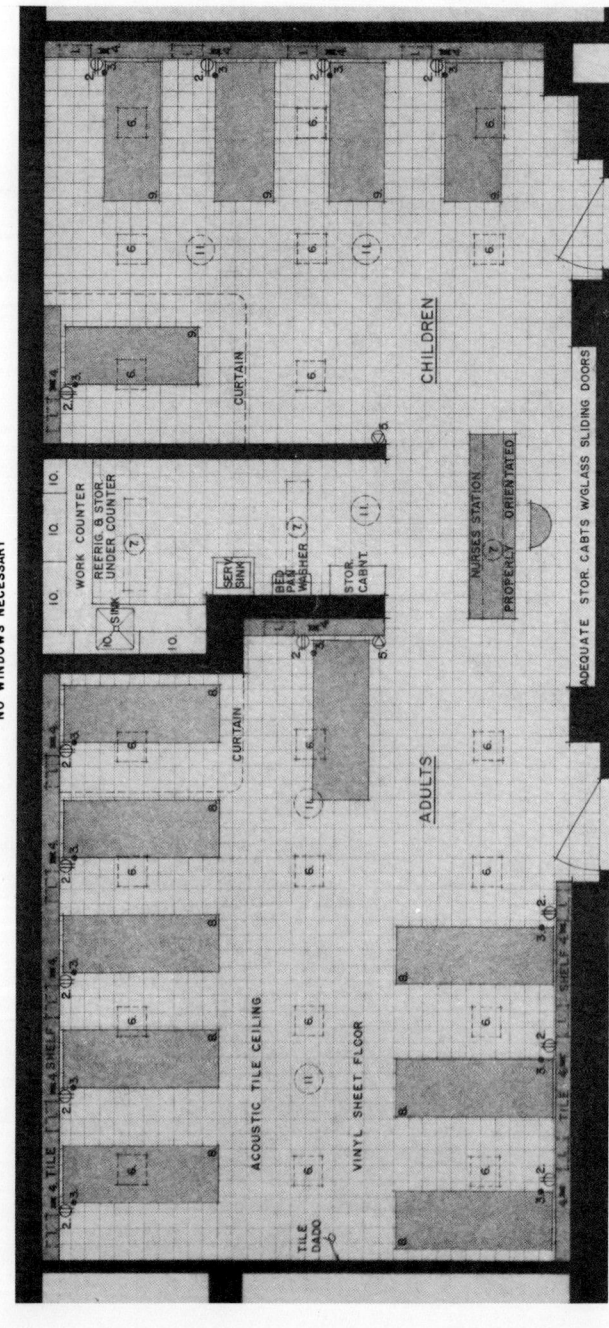

LEGEND

1. OXYGEN & 2 VACUUM OUTLETS IN RECESSED S/S CABINET
2. DUPLEX ELEC. OUTLET
3. I.V. STAND
4. BLOOD PRESSURE GAUGE
5. X-RAY OUTLET 208V
6. RECESSED OVERHEAD INCANDESCENT LIGHTING FOR COLOR
7. OVERHEAD FLUORESCENT FIXTURE FOR ADEQUATE LIGHTING
8. ADULT BED
9. CHILDRENS BED
10. LOCKABLE MEDICATION CABINETS
11. AIR CONDITIONING

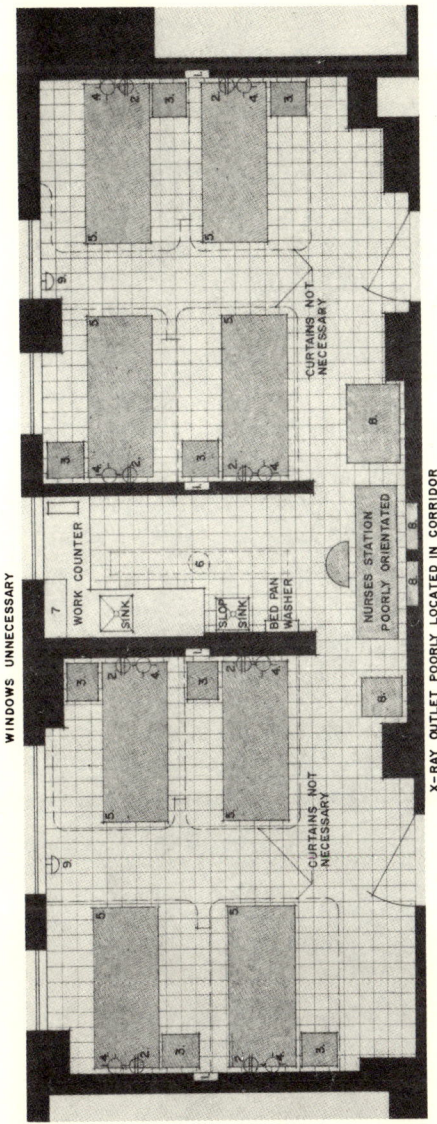

FIGURE 1
Architectural layout of a typical modern recovery room, contrasted with an earlier, less efficient version.

wish the posttonsillectomy children to be kept for varying lengths of time—in our institution, two hours—so that they may be closely observed for postoperative bleeding. We have found this procedure satisfactory. One nurse stays in the children's room, which may have four to six patients. Although they have recovered from the anesthesia and have regained their senses, they require comforting and a little TLC. If anything untoward occurs, such as large-scale vomiting or swallowing of blood that is later vomited, trained personnel are immediately available. Such situations are much easier to handle in the recovery room than when the children have returned to the pediatric wards to the care of nurses who, however well trained, are so occupied that they cannot give the very close attention required during the recovery period. We have found that care in the recovery room area requires less personnel than when the children are scattered in the pediatric division, and is otherwise more efficient.

Physical Arrangements

The general principle of having everything under direct observation should not be violated. Oxygen and suction tubes should be piped along the peripheral walls of the recovery room, with individual outlets for each patient. This is best done with a wall offset that also provides a continuous shelf upon which can be placed items required for the care of the patient. An arrangement where the patients' heads are toward the center of the room, with hanging overhead outlets, is not practicable. The nurse then looks at the back of the patients' heads, the outlets will be hazardous to tall personnel, and care will be more difficult.

Patients should be placed so that their heads are against the peripheral walls; thus, it is easier for the nurse to see the patient's face and make direct observations. The patient can also see the nurse, which is more reassuring than looking at a blank wall.

Depending upon the hospital and its equipment, the patients may be placed on special stretchers, on litters with removable sides, or on beds. We have found it preferable to have the patients remain on litters from the time they leave their rooms until they are returned to them. The orderlies who bring the patients to the operating room transport them on stretchers with sides, which are comfortable and steer and roll easily on large wheels. They should have arrangements for poles for infusion stands and brakes for locking the wheels. Immediately following the operation, the patients are placed on the same stretchers and brought to the recovery room, where they remain on their stretchers until they are discharged back to their wards. Most hospitals have acquired equipment and beds of many varieties over the years, as needed. These beds are cumbersome to move from rooms to the operating room, since they are much wider than stretchers; it would be impossible, because of the variety of types of beds, for us to keep the patient in his own bed throughout this period. Although this might theoretically be better, in our institution it has not proved practicable.

It is important, when determining the space requirements for a recovery room, to allow for the movement of stretchers. The doors should be adequately wide. Stretchers should be spaced around the walls so as to permit attendants to move freely between them. Sufficient space should be provided so that they can be moved into and out of position conveniently without bumping into other stretchers or equipment. Naturally, the room should be well lighted, have adequate electrical outlets, and in general conform to good hospital standards.

HEAT REGULATION

Temperature control in this area is important. The recovery room should be air-conditioned for patient and personnel comfort. Patients may lose large amounts of fluids through perspiration if the room is allowed to become too warm, especially during the summer. A central conditioning unit for the entire wing is best; if this is not available, the recovery room should be air-conditioned with window units. The air-conditioning system should be so arranged that the cold air is generally and evenly distributed throughout the room and not blown more on one patient close to it than on another patient further away. The temperature should be kept in the 72°-75° range. Partially

Physical and Architectural Considerations / 25

anesthetized patients are very susceptible to cold and will respond by shivering. This is to be avoided, since it greatly increases the metabolic rate and puts an unnecessary strain on the patient. A blanket warmer should be used so that needed blankets are at the proper temperature to provide the most comfort.

The heating system should be efficient and well controlled so that an even, comfortable temperature can be maintained. Good thermostatic control of this area, independent of other areas in the building, is essential.

OXYGEN AND SUCTION

The recovery room should have full facilities for oxygen administration. This is normally done by having oxygen piped to stations at the head of each patient, delivered through a flowmeter and a humidifier to plastic disposable units such as nasal catheters, masks, bags and tracheal masks.

If a piped oxygen system is not available throughout the hospital, then a bank of tanks can be set up in the immediate vicinity of the recovery room, and a small piping system can be installed for the beds there. Having large movable oxygen tanks in the room is an archaic, cumbersome method of delivering oxygen to each patient. It is both costly and inefficient, and oxygen may not be readily available to a patient in an emergency.

At least one, preferably two, suction outlets should be available on the wall at each station.

These will be used for suctioning mucus and secretions from the patient's airway and for removing gastric contents that may be vomited; they may also be attached to Levin tubes, Miller-Abbott tubes, thoracic suction, T tubes, and various other tubes that may have been inserted into the body or its orifices by the surgeon. In many instances, in place of piped suction, new plastic, self-contained, disposable suction apparatus is available in those cases that do not require large suction pressures. Sterile disposable catheters should be used for suctioning through airways, endotracheal tubes, and tracheal cannulas. Curved metal suction tips such as commonly used during tonsillectomies should be used for oral and pharyngeal suction. Both oxygen and suction outlets should be in sufficient quantity so that one of each can be immediately and continuously connected at each patient position.

NURSE'S STATION

There should be a complete nurse's station with charting facilities, which should be arranged so that the nurse sitting at her desk faces the patients. It is poor practice to locate the desk against the wall so that the nurse's back is to the patients. Although paperwork should be kept to a minimum, charts must be written, and a nurse facing away from a patient may not be aware of changes in his condition. To overcome this hazard, we have developed clip boards that, hung over

Physical and Architectural Considerations / 27

the rail of each stretcher, hold the patient's chart and the recovery room chart. In this way, any notation must be made at the foot of the patient's bed (see Figure 2). This is also more convenient for physicians visiting the recovery room; to determine the patient's condition they have only to look at the chart that is immediately visible on the clip board. This obviates the delay in asking nursing personnel to retrieve a chart from its often invisible hiding place.

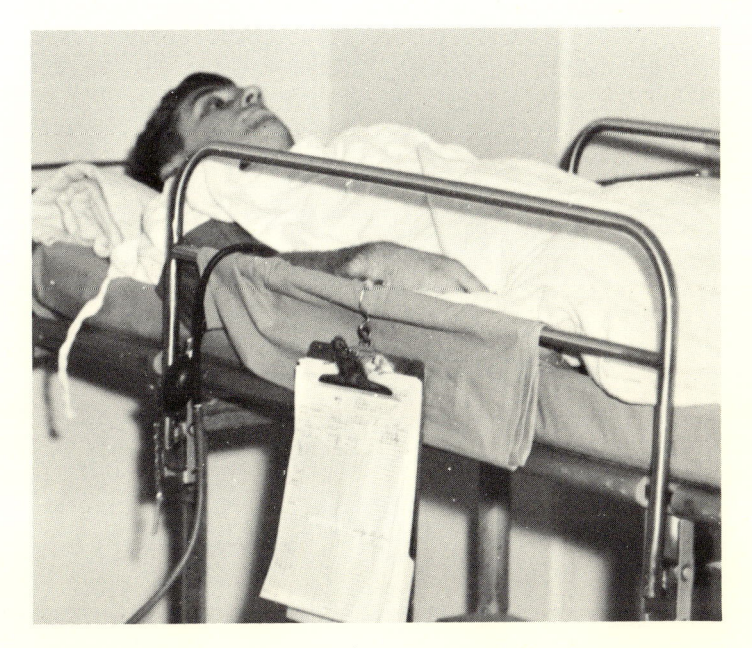

FIGURE 2
Stretcher, showing side rails and clip board arrangement for chart. The recovery room sheet is plainly visible.

28 / Manual for Recovery Room

Piping music into the recovery room may or may not be advisable. While we have no experience with it, it might prove worthwhile under sound circumstances, but soothing music rather than the type presently popular should be used.

4
EQUIPMENT

A FULL LINE of intravenous fluids and the required sets for their administration should be kept in the recovery room. A small refrigerator is useful to store blood which may be required during this period. Plasma expanders should be kept on hand for emergency use. An adequate supply of a variety of needles and syringes of the disposable variety should be kept on hand and replenished daily.

The utility room should have sinks, hoppers, and similar facilities so that soiled equipment can be cleaned in the area, eliminating the necessity for attendants to leave the recovery room. It should be a guiding principle in setting up a recovery area that it be a self-sufficient unit. As much as possible of the equipment that is required for the care of the patient should be in the recovery room, and attendants should not be required to leave the area to obtain, dispose of, or to care for equipment. Thus, minimal personnel may be used, since they will be available at all times.

Cut-down sets should be available, together with tracheotomy and thoracotomy sets (see Figure 3). A complete endotracheal tray with laryngoscopes, tubes of various sizes, and connectors should be kept handy. An assortment of various sizes of oropharyngeal airways of either the

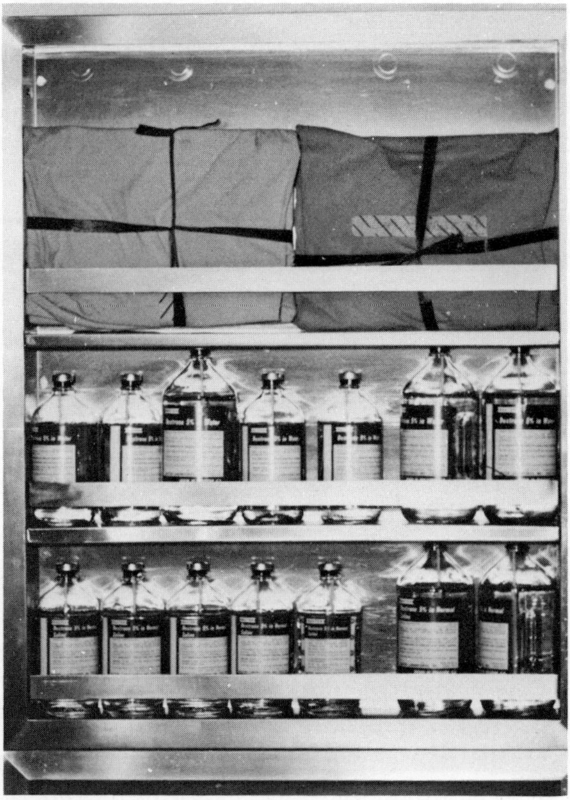

30 / Manual for the Recovery Room

FIGURE 3
Wall racks hold intravenous solutions and plainly visible tracheotomy kit and cardiac-arrest tray.

plastic or metal type should be kept on hand. Metal airways with nipples for administering oxygen are very useful and should be used when possible. All of these items must be used quickly in emergencies, and valuable time may be lost if they must be obtained from any other area. The actual contents of these sets should be determined by those who will use them; personal preferences will control the makeup of sets. The important consideration in these kits is that they be complete, plainly marked, clearly visible, and immediately available.

A means of positioning the patient should be available when stretchers, rather than beds, are used. If the stretchers are not of the type that can be adjusted to various positions, blocks or hydraulic equipment should be available so that patients may be placed either in the Trendelenburg position, when that is required, or in a Fowler's or head-up position, if this becomes necessary.

There should be adequate numbers of blood pressure cuffs and manometers, which may be put on a patient's arm and left there during his stay in the recovery room. This makes it easier and more convenient for the nurse to make frequent blood pressure determinations; if the nurse must go from bed to bed carrying a blood pressure cuff and replace it on each patient, she invariably tends to take blood pressures less frequently.

DRUG SUPPLY

A fairly extensive variety of drugs should be available. Narcotics of the types ordinarily used in the postoperative period—morphine, Pantopon, Demerol, and Nisentil—and narcotic antagonists such as Nalline and Lorfan should all be stocked.

So-called respiratory, cardiac, and central nervous system stimulants may be available, although they are infrequently used. Available information indicates that doxapram hydrochloride is an effective respiratory stimulant and should be included in the available drug armaruentarium. Vasopressor drugs, including Levophed and Aramine, must be kept on hand, although they should be used discreetly and judiciously. When first set up, the drug variety may seem quite large, but after a trial period additions, deletions, and substitutions will adjust the recovery room supply to the demands of its physicians.

MISCELLANEOUS EQUIPMENT

A mechanical means of assisting or controlling respiration should be available in the room. The simplest form of this apparatus is a bag-mask combination such as the Ambu or Hope, which can be used manually for assisting or controlling respiration, either with room air or varying amounts of added oxygen. The Bennett or Bird resuscitators and others of the intermittent positive-pressure type will perform this function automatically, but are more expensive. An active recovery room should have both of these types. The respirators can also be used to nebulize and administer such drugs as Isuprel when their use is indicated. The inhalation therapy department and its equipment are usually readily available and its members work closely with the recovery room staff, since both are normally affiliated with the anesthesia department.

In addition to having oxygen and suction available, the average recovery room should have on its shelves all the linen and supplies that are required to care for a postoperative patient. Additional dressings, changes of linen for the patients who have soiled the stretcher sheets, and the standard items required for average nursing care should be readily available. A list of these supplies should be made by the people involved and should be revised periodically. Since no list can apply to every situation, the selection should be left to the judgment of the personnel concerned. The logistics of supply vary with the hospital; individual circumstances will necessarily determine the amount of supplies that must be kept on hand to meet normal demands.

ELECTRONIC EQUIPMENT

A large amount of electronic equipment is usually not required. Monitors such as cardioscopes, pacemakers, hypothermia machines, defibrillators, and electroencephaloscopes should be acquired as desired; the amount will vary with the volume of work, the number of patients, and the complexity of the cases. The irreducible minimum is a combined unit composed of a cardioscope, a pacemaker, and a defibrillator. The accumulation of large quantities of this type of equipment will generate a space and storage problem. When the recovery room is in close proximity to the operating room, it has access to all the equipment acquired by the anesthesia department. Occasional patients may be transferred from the operating room to the recovery room still attached to such mechanical or electronic equipment as hypothermia machines or cardioscopes. Some instruction in the operation of these machines should be given to the personnel of the recovery room.

5
RESPIRATION

THE TERM respiration refers to the exchange of gases necessary to life. Two types of respiration take place in the body; internal and external. External respiration refers to the exchange of gases between the air and the blood across the alveolar membrane, while internal respiration refers to the exchange between the blood and tissue cells. The most important gases involved in this exchange are oxygen, which is taken in, and carbon dioxide, which is eliminated.

ANATOMY AND ORGANS OF RESPIRATION

The air-conducting passages consist of the nose and nasal cavity, pharynx, larynx, trachea, and bronchi. This route is followed by air as it travels from outside the body to the alveoli, where the gaseous exchange actually occurs.

Nose

The principal external organ of respiration is the nose. The surface of the nasal mucosa is covered with mucus, which is secreted continuously by goblet cells in the epithelial layer. As air passes over this wet vascular membrane, it is warmed or cooled, depending on the temperature of both the air and the patient. The nasal mucosa is covered with tiny cilia that collect dust and sweep it backward into the nasopharynx, where it is either swallowed or coughed up. Thus, the nose acts as both a humidifier and filter. Mouth breathing or tracheostomy bypasses this humidifier, and artificial humidification should be added to the inspired air.

Pharynx

The respiratory gases, after passing through the nose, enter the pharynx, which may be anatomically divided into three areas: the nasopharynx, the oropharynx, and the laryngopharynx.

The nasopharynx has a purely respiratory function, and the nasal mucosa and cilia are continuous throughout it. During the act of swallowing, the soft palate is raised by various muscles, and the nasopharynx is shut off, preventing the passage of food or fluids into it.

The oropharynx extends from the soft palate to the hyoid bone, where it joins the inferior portion of the pharyngeal cavity, the laryngopharynx. The oropharynx and the laryngopharynx serve two purposes; respiration and digestion. The blood, nerve, and muscle supplies to this area are abundant. The muscles used in the act of swallowing and in maintaining oropharyngeal posture are small in size and are markedly affected by the muscle-relaxant effects of general anesthesia. The combination of poor oropharyngeal muscle tone, which accompanies almost all general anesthetics, plus the rolling back of the tongue, may cause respiratory obstruction. The patient with poor muscular tone in the oropharynx occasionally needs support in the form of pressure anteriorly on the angle of the jaw, which puts the muscles in the oropharynx and laryngopharynx on the stretch, a position closer to normal.

Larynx

The larynx is located at the superior end of the trachea and just anterior to the laryngopharynx. It is triangular in shape and composed of nine cartilages, making it noncollapsible. During the act of swallowing, the larynx is pulled upward and forward in such a way that the air passage is shut off, thus preventing aspiration of food or foreign material. The weakened patient or one recovering from general anesthesia has a diminution of his oropharyngeal and laryngeal reflexes, so that he tends to react too slowly, or not at all, to foreign bodies in the throat, which makes aspiration of these foreign bodies more probable in these situations.

Laryngospasm is a sudden violent contraction of the vocal cords, which may or may not result in complete respiratory obstruction. Partial laryngospasm is made obvious by a "crowing" sound as air passes over and between the semiclosed vocal cords. Complete laryngospasm with total respiratory obstruction has no sound because of the absence of moving air. Complete laryngospasm progresses rapidly to anoxia and cyanosis and requires immediate attention.

Trachea

The trachea is approximately 11 cm in length and serves as the passageway between the larynx and lungs. It is located in front of the esophagus and is composed of U-shaped cartilages that prevent collapse, keeping it open at all times. The ciliated mucous membrane resumes; however, the cilia now sweep particles up to the pharynx, where again they are either swallowed or coughed up. This is the reason gastric content smears may show cells from pulmonary disorders.

Bronchial Tree

The trachea ends at the carina, where it divides into the right and left main stem bronchi. The cartilages and ciliated mucous membrane are continuous with the bronchi, although the cartilage becomes smaller and smaller as the bronchus continues and divides. The bronchi and bronchioles contain many smooth muscle fibers, which circumvent the bronchus and enable it to expand and contract. Asthma represents a condition of constricted bronchi caused by spasm and is characterized by a sense of constriction in the chest and by dyspnea. The bronchioles continue to divide until they finally divide into the alveoli, which are tiny shelflike projections, where the actual exchange of vital gases takes place across the alveolar membrane separating the alveolar sacs from the capillaries.

MECHANICS OF RESPIRATION

As stated, there is free communication from the outside air to the alveoli and the respiratory membrane. Respiratory movements create a flow of air in and out of these passages to bring fresh air in contact with the respiratory membrane. This facilitates the exchange of gases through the different pressure gradients in air as compared to blood. The partial pressure of oxygen is higher in air than in blood; in the efforts of the gas to equalize its pressure on each side of the alveolar wall, which is a semipermeable membrane, oxygen passes from air to blood. Carbon dioxide, which has a higher partial pressure in blood than in air, tends to move through the alveolar wall into the air. If the air were not changed, the partial pressures would in time tend to become equal, with the rate of flow decreasing until the pressures were equalized. Therefore, in order to keep a constant flow of oxygen and carbon dioxide in opposite directions at the alveolar membrane, it is necessary continually to bring new supplies of air into contact with the alveolar membrane.

This continuous exchange is accomplished by the respiratory movements of alternate inspiration and expiration. Inspiration is an active effort bringing a variety of muscle contractions into play, while expiration is largely passive, with relaxation of these muscles and their return to the resting state.

Inspiration

The thorax is a closed cage surrounding the lungs, which communicate with the outside air through the passages already described. The contraction of the muscles of respiration increases the size of the thoracic cage. The diaphragm descends upon contraction, increasing the vertical dimension of the thoracic cavity. The intercostal muscles elevate the ribs and tilt the sternum, increasing the anterior-posterior diameter. The lower ribs also move outward, increasing the lateral diameter of the thorax. This increase in size of the thoracic cage causes air to rush in through the communicating passages from the outside atmosphere to fill the alveoli so that the lungs can expand to fill the space created by the enlargement of the thoracic cage. This is inspiration.

Expiration

Expiration occurs as all these stretched muscles relax and return to their resting state. This recoil decreases the size of the thoracic cavity, reduces the size of the lungs, and causes air to move from the lungs to the outside.

Pleural Cavity

The pleural space is a potential space that in the normal individual contains a small amount of fluid. This fluid acts as a lubricant between the surface of the lungs and the interior of the thoracic cage so that they may slide easily against each other during the movements of respiration. When there is a pneumothorax (air in the pleural space) or a hemothorax (blood in the pleural space), the ability of the lung to expand in response to respiratory efforts is decreased. Both, or either, of these conditions may occur following surgical procedures in the thoracic cavity and can cause hypoxia. Special care must be given to these patients, as will be described later.

Rate of Respiration

The respiratory rate in the normal adult varies from 12 to 20 per minute, but slightly higher rates of 20 to 25 are considered normal in children. Tidal air, the volume inhaled and exhaled at each respiration, is usually about 400 to 500 cc. Minute volume, which is obtained by multiplying the tidal air by the rate per minute, constitutes a significant index of pulmonary ventilation. It is more indicative than either rate or depth alone, since it determines the actual supply of oxygen made available for diffusion.

REGULATION OF RESPIRATION

The rate and depth of respiration that constitutes pulmonary ventilation is under the control of the respiratory center in the medulla. This respiratory center is composed of both an inspiratory center and an expiratory center. These centers are stimulated by a multitude of impulses carried by afferent fibers and act through efferent fibers passing to the muscles of respiration.

During inspiration, the stretching of the lung tissue stimulates sensitive sensory nerve endings, which send impulses to the center. When sufficient numbers of these have been received, the muscular activity creating inspiration ceases, and expiration begins. This interaction is called the Hering-Breuer reflex and gives rise to the rhythmicity of respiration.

Respiration is also controlled by various chemical factors that act directly on the respiratory center. An increase in the carbon dioxide content of the blood stimulates respiration, especially in the presence of hypoxia. A marked decrease in carbon dioxide, as after hyperventilation, may produce decreased respiration or even a short period of apnea. Diminished oxygen levels in the blood act on the chemoreceptors in the carotid body and tend to increase respiration. The levels must be markedly reduced to produce any significant effect. Other stimulation in various parts of the body may affect respiration. Painful stimuli often produce an increase in either rate or depth. The inhalation of irritating or noxious fumes may inhibit both the rate and depth of respiration.

During recovery from anesthesia, our attention should be directed to aiding the patient to maintain an adequate rate and depth of respiration by mechanical means if his own homeostatic mechanisms have been impaired by his exposure to anesthesia and surgery.

PRACTICAL CONSIDERATIONS

The patient coming from the operating room to the recovery room has experienced some interference with his respiratory system. If he has had spinal anesthesia, its height has probably paralyzed some of the intercostal muscles and decreased his ability to expand the thoracic cage. Those who have had general anesthetics must overcome the depression of the anesthetic, possibly the lingering effects of relaxants, and perhaps the depression of preoperative narcotic medication. They may also have lost large amounts of blood, which may not have been adequately replaced. These factors may all create the problem of anoxia, or hypoxia, in the recovery room.

Anoxia

For purposes of discussion and to differentiate the various causative factors and their underlying physiology and pathology, anoxia may be arbitrarily divided into four types, depending on the etiology: (1) anoxic anoxia; (2) anemic anoxia; (3) stagnant anoxia; and (4) histotoxic anoxia.

Anoxic Anoxia

Anoxic anoxia is the inability of the patient to provide an adequate supply of oxygen to the blood at the respiratory membrane. There are several ways in which this may occur. First, respiratory obstruction may occur at any point in the pulmonary tree. We assume that the patient is in his normal environment, breathing room air that would, under normal conditions, provide an adequate supply of oxygen. The most common cause of respiratory obstruction, starting from the room air and working inward, would occur in the partially conscious patient, or the still anesthetized patient, whose tongue falls back against the pharynx and thus occludes the air passage. Further along the larynx, edema may be a cause of obstruction, either on an allergic basis or, more commonly, associated with the use of an endotracheal tube that has been malpositioned or been irritating for any period of time. A variety of irritating factors may cause a laryngospasm, wherein the patient involuntarily and reflexly closes his vocal cords and prohibits the passage of air. There may be, in addition, vomitus of a fluid or solid nature that has not been expelled from the mouth and pharynx and that may occlude the larynx. The lungs and the major bronchi may also be barriers to normal respiration. Bronchospasm, possibly caused by an asthmatic attack or by a reflex from some irritating mechanism, may constrict the passageway. Gastric contents may have been inhaled and passed into the bronchi, bronchioles, or alveoli. In the alveoli themselves there may be pulmonary edema or secretion of fluids that may interfere with the gaseous interchange by not allowing the air to come into contact with the alveolar membrane.

Narcotics and other sedatives given in the preoperative period may depress respiration by their central actions, as may anesthetic agents not completely worn off. Through central effects these depressants may depress respiration and lessen body responses to hypoxic stimuli. Muscular relaxants used during anesthesia may not have completely worn off and may interfere with the muscular efforts of respiration to such an extent that hypoxia may result.

All these causative factors of anoxic anoxia, by definition, interfere with the passage of air from the outside atmosphere through the respiratory tree to the alveolar wall, where they may come in contact with the blood. There may be mechanical or physiological obstruction at any point along this route.

Anemic Anoxia

This term obviously means that, even though an adequate supply of oxygen may reach the alveolar wall, there is insufficient circulating hemoglobin in the blood to pick up quantities of oxygen adequate to oxygenate the tissues. This may occur in patients who are either preoperatively anemic or who have lost large quantities of blood during the operative procedure.

Stagnant Anoxia

In this group, even though there is adequate oxygen coming to the alveolar wall and sufficient circulating hemoglobin to pick it up, the circulation is failing and the heart, the pump that normally circulates the blood through the lungs and thence onward through the various organs of the body, is not able to do so. The circulating time is increased, and heart failure ensues. The source of supply is adequate, and the carrier for it is available, but it is not being pumped adequately, and the stagnation of the blood produces stagnant anoxia.

Histotoxic Anoxia

Histotoxic anoxia occurs when the cells themselves have been poisoned so that, even though an adequate supply of oxygen is being delivered, the cell itself is unable to use this oxygen fully. To a small extent, this is true following most general inhalation anesthetics, but usually it is not of sufficient intensity to be clinically important.

This discussion and brief description of the types of anoxia and their etiology show how they may all be related to the patient in the recovery room following both anesthetic and surgical procedures. Considering the types in reverse order, histotoxic anoxia is not of major importance. Stagnant anoxia will be quite obvious from an evaluation of the patient's general medical and surgical condition. The diagnosis of circulatory failure should be relatively simple, and the treatment consists of cardiac supportive measures. At the same time, the inhalation of increased quantities of oxygen would be helpful so that a maximum amount would be carried to the cells, even with the slowed circulation. Anemic anoxia and the air hunger associated with it should be adequately and quickly treated by blood replacement.

Coping with these three types of anoxia, although of vital importance to the patient and at times requiring strenuous corrective measures, should not be part of the training of the recovery room personnel, who should not undertake to treat them. They require active physician participation. It is important that recovery room personnel be aware of their existence so that they may call an anesthesiologist when they occur. However, the anoxic anoxia related to the immediate mechanics of respiration and the passage of air and oxygen to the lungs is one of the major areas in which adequate nursing care can aid the patient recovering from the effects of an anesthetic.

RESPIRATORY OBSTRUCTION

The complication most frequently encountered in the recovery room is respiratory obstruction, usually mechanical in nature and located in the upper respiratory tract. In its simplest, incomplete form we have noisy respiration, such as that heard with snoring. The normal sleeping person will instinctively compensate for snoring. However, in the anesthetized or partially anesthetized patient, this slight partial obstruction may lead to a subclinical hypoxia that, if allowed to continue, may suddenly precipitate a collapse. In the more pronounced form of obstruction, the tongue may fall back against the pharynx and completely occlude the respiratory passage. Whereas snoring and noisy respiration represent vibration of tissue in the passage of air, they indicate the passage of some air. However, when the tongue falls back and completely occludes the oropharyngeal tract, the airway becomes completely obstructed and the patient makes no sound. To the inexperienced it may still seem that the patient is breathing, since there is thoracic and abdominal movement. However, these movements are occurring inversely. In the attempted inspiration, the diaphragm descends, pulling the chest in and protruding the abdomen; this paradoxical respiratory effort is completely ineffectual. The resulting asphyxia is an emergency and must be treated immediately.

Extension of the head is the position of choice in the unconscious patient. In the majority of cases this will automatically provide a patent airway. If any degree of obstruction exists, the simplest treatment, which should not await cyanosis, is to elevate the patient's jaw. Sometimes merely holding the chin up will prove effective. At other times it is necessary to grasp the angle of the jaw, one hand on each side, and elevate the entire lower jaw toward the ceiling (see Figure 4). This will usually open the air passage by elevating the base of the tongue so that the patient can breathe. If the patient is still obstructed and unable to maintain an open air passage, an oral airway should be inserted. Personnel in charge of the recovery room should be instructed in how atraumatically to insert the oropharyngeal airway (see Figure 5).

Normal respiration should be quiet, easy, and relatively deep, with very easy passage of air into

Respiration / 49

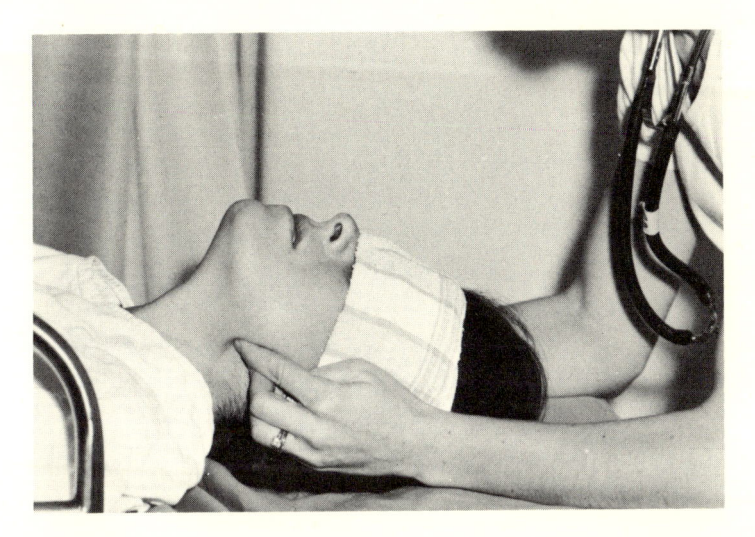

FIGURE 4
Elevating angle of jaw to raise the base of the tongue and open the air passage.

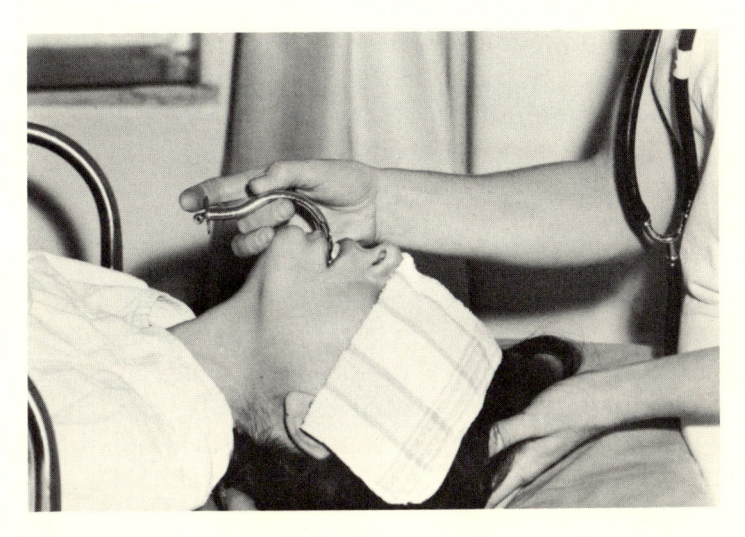

FIGURE 5
Proper method of inserting airway.

and out of the lungs. This can be checked by holding the chin up or by placing a hand very close to the patient's nose and mouth; the passage of air will then become evident. This is the easiest way to check on a patient who has obstructive breathing and in whom violent and strenuous efforts by both the thorax and the abdomen produce neither inspiration nor expiration. If there is inadequate air exchange in relation to the respiratory effort expended, even though there is not noisy breathing, some form of respiratory obstruction exists. At this time the patient may show an elevated blood pressure, and his pulse may slow. If this is allowed to progress, the patient will become cyanotic.

The Role of Artificial Airways

An airway or an endotracheal tube should not be removed from the patient until he is awake and makes some effort to remove it himself. When a patient is awake and resents the presence of an airway, it should be removed, particularly in persons in whom it causes gagging, retching, or discomfort. Usually, when the patient starts swallowing, it is time to remove the airway. After removing the airway, it is always advisable to have it immediately available for replacement if the patient becomes obstructed and does not have adequate respiratory exchange; this also applies to endotracheal tubes. If the patient is in such straits that he must come from the operating room to the recovery room with an endotracheal tube in place, he should be the one to remove it. The patient should not have been so deeply anesthetized that a prolonged period passes before he may dispense with the tube. At times it is possible to remove the endotracheal tube and replace it with an oropharyngeal airway. In any event, these tubes should not be removed until the patient starts to resent their presence, as evidenced by bucking or coughing attempts, and until there is no further danger of aspiration.

Secretions may play a part in respiratory obstruction. In some instances they may be caused by the operative procedure, especially when the operative site is intraoral or in an area that communicates with the oropharyngeal space. Obstruction may be caused by accumulation of normal secretions in the patient during a prolonged operative period, or secretions may be stimulated by the anesthetic agent. In any event, be it either blood, pus, or saliva, the fluid itself can interfere with normal respiration. If irritating and aspirated, the fluid may cause reflex bronchoconstriction and bronchospasm, followed by respiratory insufficiency. Pneumonitis, pneumonia, and atelectasis are late complications of aspiration.

RESPIRATION AND VENTILATION

The most important respiratory problems encountered in the immediate postoperative period in the recovery room are hypoventilation, airway obstruction, aspiration, and atelectasis. These lead to a reduction in respiratory efficiency, and oxygen desaturation of the arterial blood may occur.

Hypoxia and Bronchoconstriction

The earliest signs of hypoxemia and carbon dioxide retention are anxiety, restlessness, mental confusion, and hypertension. This picture should not be confused with that of pain. Unfortunately, too many physicians, seeing a patient in the immediate postoperative period restless, complaining, and thrashing about, immediately prescribe medication with an opiate. This compounds the felony; the sedation leads to more respiratory depression and more hypoxia. Instead, oxygen should be given in an attempt to overcome the hypoxia, and vigorous efforts should be made to determine the cause and correct it. This is of the utmost importance. Correction of the hypoxia will bring an immediate change in the patient and eliminate the symptoms; medication with opiates will intensify the symptoms and lead to a deterioration in the patient's condition. Patients who have decreased myocardial reserve may develop severe cardiac arrythmias with a mild hypoxia that, in other patients, might not cause any change. The patient should be made to take deep breaths and be given oxygen, and an attempt should be made to overcome the cause of the respiratory depression. Fortunately, the causes of hypoventilation are generally self-limiting and will themselves stimulate the patient to breathe deeply to correct them.

Some patients cannot increase their ventilation in sufficient amount to overcome the hypoxia and thus may experience an increase in respiratory acidosis, hypoxia, and eventual respiratory collapse. This is especially true in the older age group and in those people who have an impaired respiratory reserve before operation. They may have bronchitis, bronchoconstriction, emphysema, fibrosis, bronchiectasis, or other conditions that may interfere with normal respiratory exchange. In such cases, respiration should be assisted mechanically (see Figure 6).

Hypoxia may also be caused by pain, especially from an upper abdominal incision, which prevents or restricts the patient from taking deep

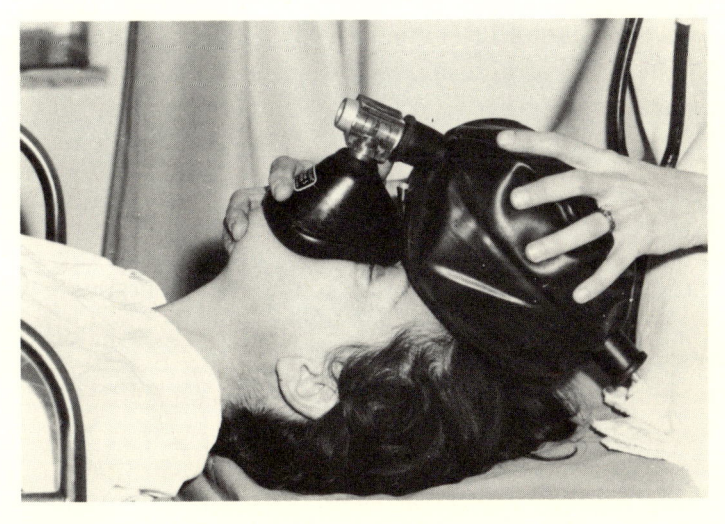

FIGURE 6
Assisting respiration with an Ambu bag.

breaths. Since the increased respiratory effort causes pain at the site of the incision, such patients will voluntarily restrict their respiratory excursions and, as a result, have limited exchange. This is also true of obese patients who, because of the effort involved, will hypoventilate. Very tight binders and dressings that restrict movements of the thoracic cage or of the abdomen should not be used. These may mechanically prevent deep breathing and proper lung expansion even if the patient attempts to breathe normally.

Bronchoconstriction may occur in the immediate postoperative period in patients who have a history of asthma or allergies. The diagnosis is made by the pronounced wheezing and increased respiratory effort with diminished exchange. Such cases should be given aminophyllin intravenously, hydrocortisone intravenously, or Isuprel nebulized through an oxygen inhalation unit. These treatments usually prove effective and relieve the bronchospasm.

Patients who have had operative procedures during which they have been paralyzed by the use of the curarizing drugs should be watched very carefully. Their muscular tonus should be evaluated either by the hand-squeezing or the head-lifting test. This is done by asking the patient to squeeze one's hand to see how much strength he has or by asking him to lift his head off the stretcher. Usually, ability to lift the head indicates that the paralytic drugs have worn off sufficiently to enable the patient to care respiratorially for himself. These patients should also be watched with specific regard to their respirations, the depth and adequacy of which should be determined in relation to the amount of air exchanged.

Several diagnostic aids serve to differentiate the causes of hypoventilation. An electric stimulator applied to a muscle will not elicit a normal response if there is residual curarization. Doxapram hydrochloride, a new selective central respiratory stimulant, injected at a dose of 1 to 2 mg/kg will immediately cause an increase in the rate and depth of respiration. If this occurs, one may attribute the depression to the lingering central effects of the premedication or the anesthetic agent. If they are caused by curarization, there will be stimulation, but no other result.

Respiration involves two chemical phases: the intake of oxygen and the excretion of carbon dioxide. Patients with inadequate, rapid, shallow respirations being given additional oxygen may very well keep themselves adequately oxygenated. However, their respirations may be insufficient in depth to eliminate carbon dioxide from the blood; as a result, they suffer from hypercapnia. Carbon dioxide in increased concentrations may sometimes act as an anesthetic. It is not uncommon to see patients in the recovery room who will respond to stimulus, but whose respirations are shallow and who will quickly fall back to sleep after they have been aroused. Such persons are inadequately eliminating their carbon dioxide and are suffering from its noxious depressant effects. Only deep respiration will adequately and efficiently eliminate carbon dioxide. For this reason, in the recovery room patients are continually stimulated to take five deep breaths.

Exercising the Patient

During the average operative procedure patients may breathe a mixture containing from 40 to 100 per cent oxygen. When they are moved to the recovery room—where they breathe the normal 20 per cent oxygen in the air, possibly enriched to 30 or 40 per cent by nasal catheters—they may show signs of anoxia. Under anesthesia and during the operation, the patient should be given a deep respiration or two every five minutes. This would correspond to the normal unanesthetized individual who during the day will, some ten or twelve times an hour, take a deep sigh. This prevents tiny areas of atelectasis from forming in the alveoli. These little pockets of atelectasis may later coalesce, augment themselves, and produce severe complications. In the recovery room, therefore, the patient should be stimulated and encouraged to take deep breaths.

The "stir-up" regime is an essential part of the recovery room care. This requires moving the patient, changing his position, urging him to take deep breaths, and encouraging him to cough. At the same time he is suctioned orally, nasally, and nasopharyngeally to remove all secretion. This stir-up regime is extremely important in returning the patient to normal functioning, particularly in regard to his respiratory system.

This is a radical change from the days when patients were kept as quiet as possible in the immediate postoperative period. One should not fear that the incision will burst when the patient is moved; it will not do so. The patient should be stimulated to move his arms and legs, to breathe deeply, and to cough.

6
CIRCULATION

ANATOMY AND PHYSIOLOGY

By maintaining a flow of blood to the various organs and tissues, the circulatory system supplies them with oxygen and nutrients and relieves them of the waste products of metabolism. It is so adaptable that, at times of stress or heightened activity, it can supply a greater blood flow to accommodate the increased metabolic activity of the local areas involved.

Heart Function

The heart provides the power to maintain the circulation, pumping the blood with sufficient pressure to propel it through the vascular system. This pressure serves three purposes: it moves the blood through the circulatory bed; it overcomes the resistance to flow and the friction of passage along the blood vessels; and it provides the filtration pressure to form the tissue fluids in the body and for glomerular filtration in the kidneys for the formation of urine.
 The heart provides the pumping mechanism for two systems: the pulmonary circulation and the general systemic circulation. The right heart pumps venous blood through the lungs, where it is

oxygenated and carbon dioxide is released. It returns to the left heart, whence it is pumped into the aorta and to the rest of the body to deliver the oxygen and take on the carbon dioxide and other waste products of metabolism.

The heart is a muscular organ with an integral impulse conduction system that stimulates the rhythmic and synchronized contraction of its four chambers. These conducting fibers start at the sinoauricular node in the right atrium and spread through the heart. The rate at which these impulses are discharged determines the heart rate, which normally may be modified by chemical changes in the blood, by temperature, and by the cardiac nerves. The origination of these impulses and their transmission may be picked up electrically; the tracing thus obtained is called the electrocardiogram.

Blood Vessels and Blood Pressure

The blood vessels may be divided into three types by their location and function. The high-pressure system of arteries and arterioles leaving the heart carries the oxygenated blood to the tiny capillaries, where the gaseous and metabolic products pass to and from the blood and tissues. Finally, the blood passes into the low-pressure collecting system, composed of venules and veins, which returns the blood to the heart.

The blood in the arteries is always under a pressure that can be measured. The unit of measurement is the height to which the pressure would support a column of mercury. The peak pressure occurring during ventricular contraction, or systole, is the systolic pressure. During ventricular relaxation, or diastole, the pressure is at its minimum value and is called the diastolic pressure. The pulse pressure is the difference between the systolic and diastolic pressures and is felt by palpation of any major artery. The pressures are maintained by the muscular wall of the arteries, which provides the necessary elasticity. In normal young adults the systolic pressure is about 120 mm of mercury and the diastolic pressure about 80 mm. The pulsations are produced by the heart; acting as a pump, it forces blood into the arteries, which then stretch under tension and are under higher pressure. The elastic recoil of these vessels pushes the blood along into the smaller arteries and arterioles. Most of this pressure is lost in forcing the blood along, into, and through the capillaries into the veins, where the pressure is from 12 mm to less than 0 mm of mercury in the vena cava.

This arterial pressure is usually measured indirectly with a sphygmomanometer. The principle is to apply external air pressure, measured by a gauge, to the arm and brachial artery and note the pressure at which the systolic and diastolic pressures are balanced. This is determined by the appearance and then disappearance of an audible beat or pulsation, as heard in the stethoscope. This is the method almost universally used to measure blood pressure.

Blood pressure is influenced by a number of

factors such as cardiac output, resistance to blood flow, the capacity of the closed vascular system, the blood volume, the viscosity of the blood, and the elasticity of the arterial system. It is readily understandable that variations in these factors may result in changes in the blood pressure. The most important of these in controlling the pressure are the regulation of the heart rate, which directly affects the cardiac output; the control of the resistance to flow; and the maintenance of the blood volume.

The heart is innervated by the vagus nerves, which are part of the parasympathetic system, and by the cardiac accelerator nerves of the sympathetic system. Stimulation of the vagus nerves slows the heart rate and reduces cardiac output per minute. Stimulation of the cardiac accelerator nerves releases norepinephrine, which increases the heart rate and thus increases cardiac output.

Resistance to blood flow is determined by the caliber of the arterioles, which can be changed by the action of the vasomotor nerves on the elastic fibers of the walls. The vasoconstrictor and vasodilator fibers are constantly active and balanced under the control of medullary centers. Stimulation of the vasoconstrictor fibers decreases the size of the arterioles, thereby shrinking the size of the vascular bed, increasing the resistance to flow, and raising the blood pressure.

The constant interplay of all these factors, the response to stimuli from various receptors, and the attempts to counteract any reactions that upset the homeostasis compose the picture of the maintenance of blood pressure.

PRACTICAL CONSIDERATIONS

For our purposes, the circulatory system can now be reduced to its simplest form and considered as a pumping system involving three basic factors. The heart is a pump; the blood is the fluid it pumps; and the system through which it pumps is composed of the arteries, capillaries, and veins. There may be derangements or troubles in any one of these three divisions. The patient may be in trouble if there is something wrong with his heart as a pump, that is, if it beats ineffectually or with disturbances in rhythm or if it is unable to perform its work as, for instance, in valvular disease or a myocardial infarction. In the recovery room, patients who have disturbances in their blood volume from blood loss that has not been adequately replaced during the operative procedure may show hypotension. There may be disturbances in the vascular bed that may affect the ability of the heart to pump the blood adequately through this circulatory system. The maintenance of circulation is dependent upon the cardiac output, and this in turn is dependent upon the return circulation to the heart. Affecting this is the peripheral resistance, which varies with the tone and state of the peripheral vascular bed. When failure occurs it may be central, that is, of the heart itself, or peripheral, as a failure in the vascular bed.

Effects of Anesthesia

The anesthetics and many of the drugs used in preoperative medication are cardiovascular depressants. These drugs decrease the ability of the body to accommodate and compensate for such alterations as blood loss and changes in the position of the patient. Bleeding during the operative procedure will, if in small amounts, be automatically compensated for by the body's ability to vasoconstrict the peripheral vascular bed and decrease its volume. In this manner the volume of blood needed is diminished, and the status quo may be maintained. Hypovolemia is a reduction in the volume of circulating blood. This occurs when there is a period of either rapid, slow, or steady loss of blood that has not been replaced. The blood pressure in these patients may be normal, but there is usually a tachycardia. It is more important to be concerned about a rapid pulse rate of over 120 per minute than about the blood pressure. Patients exhibiting this tachycardia have reduced cardiac efficiency and relatively inefficient coronary blood flow.

During anesthesia with high concentrations of oxygen, shallow respiration will maintain oxygenation of the patient; however, carbon dioxide may accumulate if respiration is not assisted. The carbon dioxide may produce vasoconstriction of the peripheral circulation and maintain the blood pressure, thus masking impending shock during the operative procedure. When the operation terminates and the anesthetic is stopped, rapid elimination of the carbon dioxide may precipitate a collapse. At this time the patient is breathing oxygen concentrations reduced below the level he received during the operation. He quickly eliminates the accumulated carbon dioxide. This is frequently evident after inadequate ventilation during cyclopropane anesthesia and is called cyclopropane shock. However, it may occur with any anesthetic agent when carbon dioxide is allowed to accumulate in large amounts that are rapidly eliminated when use of the anesthesia machine and rebreathing absorber is discontinued.

When the operation has been concluded, great care must be taken in moving the patient from the operating table to the stretcher. As already mentioned, the vascular stabilizing mechanisms of the patient at this time are not as effective as they are in the unanesthetized patient. Rough and traumatic handling of the patient may precipitate a sudden hypotension or collapse. It is very important that the patient be handled most gently with adequate personnel so that the movement may be slow and gentle. If the patient is not in good condition, if the pulse and blood pressure are not within relatively normal ranges, it is wise to keep the patient on the table until he has been stabilized. If this is not done, the recovery room may be presented with a patient in severe hypotension or shock.

Moving and Initial Care of the Patient

It must be remembered that patients coming to the recovery room and emerging from the anesthesia may struggle, thrash about, and be very restless because of pain or hypoxia, or both. Such patients have had respiratory and myocardial depressors as anesthetics. Opiates or narcotics given for relief of pain are also depressants. Since the underlying cause of the restlessness may be hypoxia, before any sedatives are administered the patient should be given an oxygen-enriched atmosphere to breathe; this may bring dramatic relief from the restlessness. If pain is the actual cause, small doses of narcotics may be given, in half the amounts usually considered adequate in the postoperative period. This half-dose routine should be established as a policy and varied only in unusual cases. It is better to give small amounts and repeat them if necessary than to give a large dose, which may result in unwarranted and severe depression of the patient.

SHOCK

Shock is a peripheral vascular failure phenomenon in which there is a disparity between the peripheral circulatory bed and the circulatory volume. It may be due to a variety of contributory causes such as toxicity, trauma, adverse neurogenic or psychogenic stimuli, and excess loss of blood, fluids and electrolytes. It tends to become irreversible if allowed to continue. Some cardinal signs of shock are pallor, clamminess of the skin, hypotension, tachycardia, evidence of vasoconstriction, and altered respirations, which may be rapid, shallow, and depressed, with signs of air hunger. Usually there is restlessness and the patient may show anxiety, apathy, or unconsciousness. Thirst is commonly seen.

When the body is first subjected to the stimuli or the causes that produce shock, it automatically compensates by trying to counteract these causes. There is an outpouring of epinephrine, which produces a rise in the systolic blood pressure by causing peripheral vasoconstriction, thereby diminishing the size of the vascular bed. An increase in the pulse rate results in an increase in cardiac output. The body also attempts to increase the circulating volume by shifting fluids from the extracellular spaces into the blood. The pulse accelerates in an attempt to increase the circulating minute volume. The cerebral and coronary vessels dilate to increase the availability of oxygen to these organs. If these compensatory mechanisms are inadequate to maintain homeostasis, deterioration occurs. The patient begins to lose quantities of fluid by sweating; the vessels that had constricted may start to dilate and leak fluids into the interstitial spaces, thus further diminishing the circulating blood volume. Very severe tachycardia may diminish the coronary blood flow and also the cardiac output; the deterioration now becomes progressive, and the patient pursues a downhill course.

Causes of Shock

Three main factors may cause shock during

surgery and in the recovery room: hemorrhage, neurogenic disturbances, and tissue trauma. These three factors are present in most surgical interventions, and all are important in realizing the mechanisms, diagnosis, and treatment of shock. The role of hemorrhage is easily understood. There is a loss of blood; an inability of the body to compensate, especially when the loss is rapid; and a diminution in the circulating blood volume. If the blood loss is slow and continuous, the body can compensate by hemodilution. However, in rapid blood loss the body does not have time to pull fluid from the tissues, and the reduction in circulating blood volume may produce shock.

Neurogenic factors may also be called the patient's reaction to stress. Frequently patients who have relatively minor traumatic injuries but who are very nervous and apprehensive due to a psychotraumatic experience may show signs of shock, unless they are handled gently and carefully. This is a psychogenic problem. Tissue damage may result in a shocklike picture, not because of the loss of fluids, but because of the release of some substance from traumatized tissues that has a deleterious effect on vascular integrity and on the body's ability to compensate.

Diagnosis of Shock

Diagnosis depends on a combination of signs and symptoms that point to a state of peripheral circulatory collapse. Of importance in this diagnosis are the condition of the skin; signs of cerebral dysfunction; thirst and oliguria; and pain, blood pressure, pulse, and heart rate. The skin condition is most readily observed. An early and active sign of shock is evidence of vasoconstriction from sympathetic stimulation, which often makes venipuncture exceedingly difficult. At the same time the overactivity of the sympathetic system results in sweating, which makes the skin wet. This gives rise to the description "cold and clammy." This is easily differentiated from wetness of the skin that may result from an excess of carbon dioxide. The hypercapnic skin is pink rather than pale; the veins tend to be dilated rather than constricted; and the pulse is full and bounding rather than feeble and rapid. In shock the skin is cold, pale, and wet. Cerebral dysfunction is shown by signs of anxiety, apathy, confusion, nervousness, agitation, or complete unconsciousness. Confusion is probably the best description of this state. Oliguria appears only after the condition has existed for a relatively prolonged period. The decreased blood pressure is insufficient to provide adequate filtration pressure in the kidneys. Thirst, restlessness, and tachycardia are the early signs of shock. Thirst results from the body's attempt to pull fluids from the interstitial spaces to compensate for the reduction in the circulating blood volume. The presence of pain is of little aid in the diagnosis since it is present in varying degree in all postoperative patients. Although the patient in shock may not complain of pain, this symptom in itself is of little importance in the diagnosis.

The pulse and its character are very significant in the diagnosis of shock and also as a gauge of the efficacy of the therapy and the prognosis of the condition. An increasing pulse rate and falling pulse pressure are bad prognostic signs. Increasing tachycardia is an early sign of shock. A rapid, soft, thready pulse is a later manifestation found in the patient who is failing to compensate adequately.

In general, laboratory tests are of slight aid. One specific test that may be of value when shock is due to blood loss is measurement of the circulating blood volume. This measurement will give an indication of the reduction in blood volume and of the amount required for adequate replacement. In this respect the hematocrit determination may also be of value.

Management of Shock

The central venous pressure, which should be monitored, serves as an excellent guide to effectiveness of treatment. Normal values should be from 10 to 15 cm of water. This is easily measured by adding a three-way stopcock to an intravenous setup and adding an open-ended arm such as an intravenous extension set. This extension arm is taped to an intravenous pole against a ruled scale. By putting this arm into the circuit via the stopcock, the pressure can be measured whenever desired. In order to have effective pumping action, adequate amounts of blood must be returned to the heart. The central venous pressure is an indication of return flow of blood to the heart. Replacement should be continued until the pressure has returned to within normal limits.

The prevention of shock is of the utmost importance. Prior to operation, the patient's blood picture should be brought to as normal a state as possible; fluid and electrolyte therapy should be carried out to bring the patient to the optimum condition. A patient in shock should never be subjected to an operative procedure unless failure to operate immediately would imply a further serious progression of the shock and perhaps death. Fluids should be replaced before operative intervention in patients, such as those suffering from intestinal obstruction, who have been vomiting in the preoperative period or who have had large volumes of body fluid pass into such body spaces as the peritoneal cavity or into dilated loops of bowel.

A clinical syndrome often found presents the patient who is in incipient but compensated shock. These postoperative patients have had a significant diminution in their total circulating volume, but have compensated by constriction of their peripheral vascular bed so that they present a relatively normal blood pressure. They are usually pale, with a dry skin and slightly increased respiratory rate. If handled carelessly and roughly or given large doses of narcotics, they may precipitously go into shock. The pulse is a valuable index to their therapy. Serial pulse and blood pressure determinations will show the effectiveness of the therapy. If one sees an increasing pallor and increasing tachycardia in such patients, an impending state of shock should be considered.

When possible, the treatment should be specific and directed toward elimination of the causative factors when these can be determined. When blood loss or other factors can be demonstrated, immediate action should be taken to correct the cause. Speed is very important and is the essence of all shock therapy. Blood replacement should be done as quickly as possible. If the patient has been typed and cross-matched beforehand and blood is quickly available, this should be used. The majority of patients who develop shock in the postoperative period are in need of blood replacement. It is very common for the surgical team to underestimate the amount of blood lost. If blood is not immediately available, plasma or blood expanders such as Dextran and Gentran should be used immediately in an effort to restore the circulating volume and maintain the blood pressure until such time as blood may be obtained. These expanders are not to be considered as substitutes for blood, but as temporary expedients to maintain circulation and prevent the progression of shock until more definitive therapy can be carried out.

Much work is now being done on the use of frozen stored blood. When fully developed and available to the average community hospital, this method will extend the usefulness of blood banks. Large quantities of red cells can be stored in freezers almost indefinitely, warmed and reconstituted in 20 minutes or less, and administered with little or no cross-matching. This technique will make our task easier and simplify the problems of blood replacement.

Vasopressors may also be of value in the treatment of shock. Drugs such as Levophed, Aramine, and Neo-Synephrine are very effective vasoconstrictors. They are relatively short-acting and may sufficiently decrease the size of the peripheral bed by vasoconstriction to stabilize the circulation until such time as definitive treatment can be undertaken. These vasopressors are never to be considered as substitutes for replacement of blood volume, but merely as temporizing measures. They should be given only when ordered by a physician.

More recent concepts in the treatment of shock put great emphasis on the maintenance of tissue perfusion. This is a more reasonable approach than focusing all attention on raising the blood pressure. Alpha-blocking agents such as chlorpromazine and Dibenzyline will eliminate the vasospastic effects from the adrenergic response of the body and will increase capillary blood flow and tissue perfusion. Great care must be taken, since their administration results in a tremendous increase in the capacity of the circulatory system. If measures are not already being taken to increase the circulating volume, death may ensue immediately. Lactated Ringer's solution is the fluid of choice in the immediate treatment of shock to increase the circulating blood volume. It almost exactly duplicates the composition of the extracellular fluid. Relatively large quantities can be given very rapidly.

The acidosis usually present in shock should be measured by blood pH analysis. Sodium bicarbonate is then administered intravenously in amounts adequate to bring the pH to within normal limits. Cortisone and its derivatives may also play a role in shock therapy. Today, with many people on steroid therapy for prolonged periods for the treatment of medical problems, the patient may have become dependent upon an outside source of these corticosteroids, which should be supplemented during the operative period. Oxygen should be given to these patients, since there exists a tissue hypoxia based on inadequate circulation. Therefore, as high a concentration as possible should be given as soon as feasible, and this should be continued as long as signs of shock exist. A mask rather than a nasal catheter or tent should be used.

Narcotics and sedatives should be given with great caution. A very small dose should be used, perhaps one fourth of the normal amount in a patient in shock, if there are severe complaints of pain. It must be remembered that the sensorium of these patients may be greatly disturbed and that such signs as restlessness, nervousness, and anxiety indicate shock and hypoxia that, in many instances, will disappear as compensation takes place and treatment is successful. In most instances, therefore, narcotics and sedatives should be used very sparingly, if at all.

7
EMERGENCE FROM ANESTHESIA

THERE ARE two broad classifications of anesthesia: (1) in which the patient has been put to sleep; and (2) in which he has had some form of regional anesthesia and remained awake during the operative procedure. General anesthetics—agents that render the patient unconscious—include those given by inhalation, intravenously, or rectally. The commonly used volatile inhalation agents, those that are in liquid form and are vaporized during administration, include Vinethene, ethyl chloride, ether, Fluothane, and Penthrane. Those that are supplied as gases in tanks are nitrous oxide and cyclopropane. The popular intravenous agents are sodium thiopental, Brevital, and Surital. Uncommonly used are the rectal agents such as Avertin and sodium thiopental. In addition, narcotic analgesics such as Nisentil and Demerol may be used intravenously to reinforce a weak inhalation agent. Muscle paralyzants are often used to provide relaxation during general anesthesia. This combination permits use of greatly reduced amounts of anesthetic agents. Spinal anesthetics are the regional agents most commonly used. Caudal anesthesia, nerve blocks of various types, and, most recently, intravenous perfusion of a limb have become popular. All of these agents may produce specific problems during emergence from their effects and because of the actions of other medications used with them. These will be discussed individually.

CYCLOPROPANE

The recovery from anesthesia to semiconsciousness or full consciousness is usually rapid, with little or no remaining analgesia. These patients will frequently require some sedation very early in the postoperative period. There may be some nausea and vomiting; retching is more frequent, but usually is not severe. Occasional patients may have a severe emergence delirium characterized by severe thrashing about and incoherence requiring restraint. This is not common, but may occur and should be treated with small doses of narcotics such as 25 to 50 mg of Demerol, or 1/8 grain of morphine given intravenously. This emergence delirium may be attributed to recovery from anesthesia in the presence of pain from the operative intervention.

If ventilation has not been adequate during anesthesia, patients who have been under cyclopropane with high oxygen concentrations may develop a very high carbon dioxide blood level. When the anesthesia is discontinued and this hypercapnia is rapidly eliminated, these patients may show a severe blood pressure drop. This hypotension, although it may be severe, is usually accompanied by a slow full pulse and a pink dry skin, so that even with a very low blood pressure the patient does not present the picture typical of peripheral vascular collapse. "Cyclopropane shock" is the term usually used to describe this picture. No special treatment is required, and the patients recover with no more than the usual general care.

ETHER

Recovery from ether anesthesia is much slower. Ether is much slower in induction, is deposited in the fatty tissues during administration, and is eliminated less rapidly. Patients who have had prolonged ether anesthesia will probably show some signs of acidosis, will be sweaty, and will probably vomit somewhat more than those subjected to other general inhalation anesthetics. Because of this slow elimination there is a period of analgesia while the patient is waking from the ether anesthesia. There is usually no hypotension if the fluid balance has been maintained. Increased salivation and gastric irritation may cause vomiting in the postoperative period.

HALOTHANE

Fluothane and Penthrane are the two agents most commonly used in this family of anesthetics. Fluothane has a rapid recovery time, with little or no lingering analgesia. In contrast to those given other anesthetics, these patients often look pale and may show some respiratory depression. Hypoventilation should be treated by the administration of an oxygen-enriched atmosphere via a nasal catheter or face mask. Respiration should be assisted with an Ambu or other bag-mask combination. Vocal stimulation and the stir-up regime will be especially useful here. Patients recovering from Penthrane anesthesia may show more analgesia in the postoperative period than those who have had Fluothane, but they sleep somewhat longer.

ETHYL CHLORIDE

Ethyl chloride is of no importance here since, when it is employed, it is used as an induction agent to be followed, probably, by ether. Induction and emergence are very rapid.

NITROUS OXIDE

Today, nitrous oxide is probably the most commonly used inhalation anesthetic; it is employed in conjunction with another anesthetic agent such as Pentothal, halothane, or ether, or with a relaxant. Of itself, it has minimal postanesthetic effects, and any complications in its use would be caused by associated agents. As long as hypoxia is prevented during administration, there are no systemic effects from nitrous oxide. It is rapidly eliminated, with little if any nausea, so that the patient is usually reacting on arrival in the recovery room.

NARCOTIC ANESTHESIA

Nisentil is the most frequently used narcotic for anesthesia in combination with nitrous oxide, with or without a relaxant. The patient is usually awake and responding when brought to the recovery area, with little or no excitement or restlessness. There is very good postoperative analgesia. The patient may drop back to sleep, but is easily wakened by the spoken voice and cooperates with requests. As with other anesthetics, respiration must be carefully observed for signs of depression. Deep breathing should be encouraged, and a narcotic antagonist may be used if necessary. In the dosage properly used there are no systemic effects other than respiratory depression. Usually nausea and vomiting are totally absent.

INTRAVENOUS BARBITURATES

Sodium Pentothal and the other agents in this group of barbiturates are basically hypnotics producing sleep, rather than analgesics that diminish or eliminate the sensation of pain. A sleep sufficiently profound will eliminate a reaction to painful stimuli.

Due to their ease of administration, rapidity of action, and excellent patient acceptance, barbiturates are usually used to induce sleep before the administration of other anesthetics. When used in this fashion as induction agents, their effects are dissipated by the end of the procedure. For minor procedures they are often used with nitrous oxide as a bolstering anesthetic. When used in properly balanced fashion, awakening is rapid with minimal nausea and little analgesia. At times these patients may show delirium and uncooperative thrashing, necessitating narcotics for pain relief and sedation. Again, this is probably due to the patient's being only partially awake and not in full control of his senses while he is subjected to painful stimuli.

These patients should be watched carefully for respiratory obstruction and laryngospasm. The presence of secretions or other foreign material in the oropharynx may stimulate the vocal cords, since pentothal does not dull the pharyngeal and laryngeal reflexes.

RECTAL ANESTHESIA

This route of administration is infrequently used. Its great disadvantage is a prolonged recovery time, with patients often sleeping for many hours. Rectally, drugs are slowly but continuously absorbed, and the prolonged recovery time prevents an adequate stir-up regime. These patients should have periodic respiratory assistance to ensure deep breathing and complete lung inflation at periodic intervals to prevent areas of atelectasis. Suctioning to prevent the accumulation of secretions should be done regularly.

SPINAL ANESTHESIA

Spinal anesthesia is produced by infecting a solution of a local anesthetic into the spinal fluid in the subarachnoid space, causing a temporary paralysis of sensory, autonomic, and motor fibers in the nerve roots that are bathed by the drug. The anesthesia is not caused by the drug's entering the cord itself.

Upon admission to the recovery room, the patient who has received a spinal anesthetic is usually awake unless he has been put lightly to sleep during the procedure for psychic reasons. Although these patients are awake, it is essential to ascertain that there is no excess pressure on the lower extremities at any time. The patient cannot feel his legs and therefore cannot complain about a malposition or pressure. Pressure areas leading to necrosis can develop quickly. If a position change is indicated, the patient must be turned slowly; a rapid change of position or roughness in handling will cause hypotension. The spinal anesthesia has diminished the ability of the peripheral vascular bed in the lower part of the body to compensate for changes in position.

Unless otherwise specified, the patient may

have a small pillow under his head. Keeping the head flat is very uncomfortable for the patient and probably does nothing to diminish the incidence of postspinal headache.

Spinal anesthesia for abdominal operations often results in paralysis of at least the lower half of the intercostal muscles. This eliminates the use of this part of the thoracic cage in respiration and may result in hypoxia if the other muscles of respiration are not able to compensate. This paralysis also interferes with the ability to breathe deeply and cough effectively. These patients should be observed carefully and their respiratory movements watched to determine when the descending recovery of muscular activity returns as the anesthetic wears off. Decreasing analgesia should be noted; analgesia will last from 2 to 4 hours. The patient's ability to feel when touched is the first sign that the anesthetic is wearing off. The ability to move the toes and then the feet shows almost complete recovery from anesthesia. Spinal anesthesia also causes a vasodilatory effect on the kidneys that may increase diuresis. Overdistension of the bladder is likely to occur and should be watched for, since bladder sensation is not present.

Other regional anesthetics present no problems other than those caused by absorption of the anesthetic agents. The release of the tourniquet after intravenous perfusion techniques may be followed by transient dizziness. A severe toxic reaction with collapse is treated symptomatically with a vasopressor and intravenous fluids; this is a very uncommon occurrence.

RELAXANTS

The use of muscle relaxants has become almost routine during general anesthesia for operations requiring muscular relaxation. If used only to facilitate intubation, the effects wear off within 5 minutes and are of no concern in the postoperative period. In those cases where a relaxant such as succinylcholine, tubocurarine, or gallamine is used throughout a procedure, with controlled or assisted respiration, the adequacy of the patient's ventilatory efforts must be watched carefully.

When the patient is responding, the return of muscle tone can be tested by asking the patient to raise his head or by testing the strength of his hand squeezing. Inadequacy in either of these efforts should alert the staff to hypoventilation. The diaphragm and intercostal muscles are both necessary to adequate chest expansion. If the intercostals are still paralyzed, there will be diminished chest expansion, and assistance of respiration may be required for proper elimination of carbon dioxide. Adequate oxygenation may be maintained by the addition of oxygen through the use of a nasal catheter or face mask.

8
PATIENT CARE

A DEFINITE ROUTINE should be established for the admission of patients from the operating room to the recovery room. The anesthetist must accompany the patient into the recovery room and discuss the case, however briefly, with the nurse in charge. The practice of pushing the patient into the room or through the doorway and thus transferring him to the recovery personnel should never be tolerated; the anesthetist should participate in the admission procedure.

A nine-point procedure for admission should be established as follows:

1. Receive patient from anesthetist and check for any unusual orders and procedures.
2. Make certain respirations are unobstructed and adequate.
3. Check pulse and blood pressure and record on chart.
4. Position patient; check side rails.
5. Inspect dressings; check for bleeding.
6. Check intravenous fluids for infiltration.
7. Check postoperative orders.
8. Start record for patient.
9. Start stir-up regime.

The list seems to imply that many things should be

done at once; actually, these steps all flow together and very soon become automatic. The proper routine in accepting the patient is a most important part of achieving proper patient care in the recovery room.

STIR-UP REGIME

The stir-up regime is one of the most important factors in the prevention of thoracic complications and should be an integral part of any postoperative management. It has six basic divisions:

1. <u>Cough.</u> Support the incisional area and encourage coughs of 10 to 20 seconds, depending on the amount of secretions. Oral suction with a catheter or metal tip removes the secretions and also stimulates the patient to cough.

2. <u>Deep-breathing Exercises</u>. The patient should take 6 to 10 deep breaths every 5 to 10 minutes, with close observation of depth and rate. Full inflation of the lungs prevents small areas of patchy atelectasis from developing.

3. <u>Position Changes.</u> Turn the patient from side to side and encourage him to move unaided, if possible. Care must be taken so that any drainage tubes that may be in place are not disturbed, kinked, or accidentally pulled out. This care should also be taken with the needles used for intravenous solutions.

4. <u>Mobilization.</u> The patient must be made to move his arms and legs in rhythmic fashion. This diminishes peripheral stasis and lessens the danger

of thrombosis. The exertion automatically causes deep breathing, aids venous return, and improves cardiac function.

    5. <u>Narcotics and Sedatives</u>. All narcotics depress the cough reflex and ciliary activity that help to clean out the lungs. When these cough reflexes are depressed, secretions build up, predisposing to atelectasis. In some cases, narcotics may lower alveolar ventilation to the point of causing respiratory acidosis and hypoxia, leading to harmful pulmonary capillary bed leakage into the lungs.

    6. <u>Suctioning</u>. The removal of secretions that may have accumulated in the respiratory passages is essential to maintain a clear and unobstructed airway. A soft rubber or plastic suction catheter should be inserted gently into the oropharynx and nasopharynx. Care must be taken to prevent trauma and bleeding, which may more than negate any benefits obtained from suctioning other secretions. Deep breathing should be encouraged between aspirations if the patient is awake. Patients who have not yet responded should have assisted respirations, with deep inflations after the secretions have been cleared. Do not try to hyperinflate the lungs manually if the secretions are still present because they may be forced deep into the lungs where they may not be readily accessible by suction. A Y-tube should always be installed in the suction line so that it can be used intermittently. This prevents constant suction, which might empty the air out of the lungs and cause the very atelectasis we are trying to prevent. Apparati commonly used are shown in Figure 7.

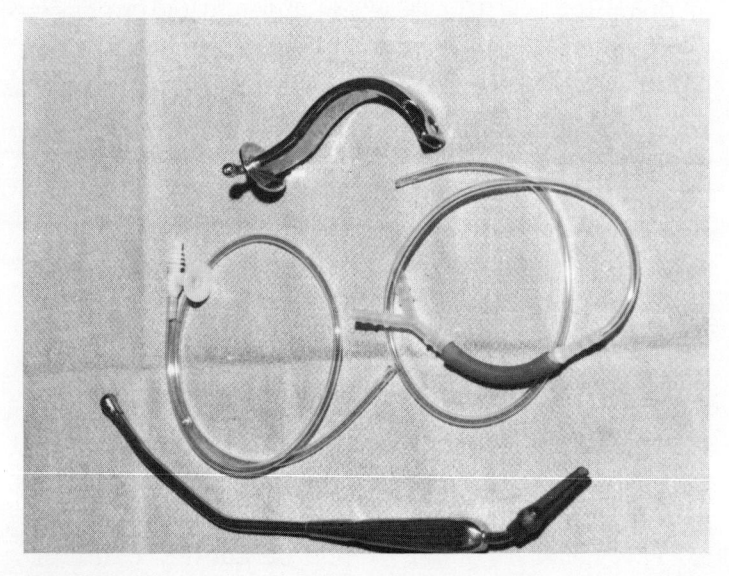

FIGURE 7
Metal tip and two catheters set up for intermittent suction.

BLOOD TRANSFUSION REACTIONS

Blood transfusion reactions may occur when only a few drops of donor's blood have been transfused; alternatively, they may be delayed as long as 24 hours after the transfusion is completed. Of concern to us in this period are those that occur and show symptomatology within several hours of administration. Reactions to blood transfusions may occur because of incompatibility or idiosyncrasies. The types of reactions are characterized as allergic, febrile, and hemolytic.

Allergic reactions are the most common. Typical signs of allergy may appear; these include skin rash, itching, and urticaria; edema of the eyes, face, and lips; and, most dangerous, edema of the uvula and laryngeal area. This edema may produce an acute respiratory obstruction that may be complete and fatal. When this type of reaction occurs, it should be treated with adrenalin, an antihistamine, or cortisone, as determined by a physician.

A febrile response is a very important sign of a blood transfusion reaction. This reaction occurs during or shortly after a transfusion. The patient's temperature may rise to from $100°$ to $104°F$ and may remain elevated for from 8 to 12 hours. This rise is often preceded by a chill of varying intensity. The chill should be treated symptomatically with hot water bottles and warm blankets.

A hemolytic reaction is caused by an increased rate of destruction of either the donor's or the recipient's red cells. Agglutination of red blood cells may occur in the smaller blood vessels and capillaries, plugging them. When these red cells are destroyed, large quantities of hemoglobin are released; these may plug the kidneys, interfering with the normal filtration system that produces urine. Complete kidney blockage followed by anuria may prove fatal.

Most of these reactions are due to incompatible blood. The postanesthesia patient who has received blood or is receiving blood should be watched carefully for such symptoms as flushed skin, rash, urticaria, fever and chills, unexplained hypotension, restlessness, tachycardia, petechiae, obstructed breathing, arrhythmic pulse, unexplained oozing of blood, and blood in the urine.

The first thing to be done when there is a possibility that a reaction is occurring is to stop the transfusion. Start saline in its place; do not remove the intravenous tube or destroy the remaining blood, which should be returned to the laboratory for checking. Call for medical help, preferably from a physician in the anesthesia department. Treat the patient symptomatically with blankets for chills and oxygen for any hypoxia. More definitive measures can be instituted by the doctor after he has appraised the situation.

HYPERTENSION IN THE IMMEDIATE POSTOPERATIVE PERIOD

A rise in blood pressure in patients previously normotensive is not uncommon. When seen in the recovery room, it may be due to a wide variety of causes. Hypertension arising during anesthesia may carry over into this period. Vasopressors given for a hypotensive state during anesthesia may be rapidly absorbed as the circulation improves. Respiratory obstruction or hypoventilation causing carbon dioxide retention, with or without hypoxia, may cause a rise in pressure. Some surgical procedures may cause a hypertension: for example, the fluid absorption syndrome after transurethral resection or a rise in intracranial pressure after neurosurgical procedures and head injuries. Other metabolic causes may be an unrecognized pheochromocytoma or a thyroid crisis after thyroidectomy. An emergence delirium with its excitement and struggling will usually cause a transient rise in pressure.

The treatment is basic and consists of determining and eliminating the cause, where possible. Unless the pressure rises to very high levels, with complaints of headache, and a cerebral vascular accident is feared, drugs such as Arfonad and Regitine should not be used. Amyl nitrite by inhalation will usually overcome a transient rise. Any drug therapy should be given only by a physician's order after he has evaluated the situation.

HYPOTENSION IN THE IMMEDIATE POSTOPERATIVE PERIOD

Postural changes such as moving the patient from table to stretcher may produce a lowering of blood pressure if the movement is rough or jerky. The typical picture of surgical shock exhibits a low pressure, as does unrecognized blood loss or inadequately treated hypovolemia during the operation. Narcotics for pain should not be given in excessive doses, and intravenous doses should not be given too rapidly. Transfusion reactions, as previously mentioned, may produce a shocklike state. Respiratory acidosis during anesthesia, followed by a rapid decrease in carbon dioxide tension, may show a hypotension associated with a slow bounding pulse. Withdrawal of high oxygen concentrations when the mask is removed may cause a lowering of blood pressure, together with hypoxia. Massive pulmonary emboli may produce a severe circulatory collapse and death.

Hypotension is a sign of some derangement in the circulatory system. It should not be treated only as a symptom, with a vasopressor given to raise the pressure. It is important that the etiology be determined and that corrective measures be taken. General measures such as use of the Trendelenburg position and oxygen administration should be instituted quickly while medical aid is being summoned.

CONTROL AND PREVENTION OF INFECTION

The recovery room personnel should take the same care in patient contact to prevent infection or cross-infection as do nurses in any other area of the hospital. It is important that those assigned to the recovery room be free of upper respiratory disease that might, through coughing or sneezing, infect those who come under their care. The common cold, so prevalent in everyday life, may be very serious when transmitted to the postoperative patient. Personnel who come in contact with patients during this critical period should be free of all respiratory infections. It goes without saying that carriers, especially of staphylococcus or streptococcus, must be barred from the recovery room. Patient contamination may result from intermediate contact with another patient. These considerations of good nursing practice should be emphasized when dealing with these very vulnerable patients; a nurse caring for one infected case and then, without precautions, caring for another relatively clean patient would violate these conventions. In general, patients who have abscesses or severe respiratory infections should be placed in a separate area of the recovery room, where they will not come into contact with other patients.

All objects that come into physical contact with one patient and may subsequently touch another should be sterilized between contacts. Principally, this involves blankets, instruments, stethoscopes, blood pressure cuffs, suction apparatuses, and face masks. The present trend toward the use of disposable equipment facilitates this task.

A gas sterilizer is very useful to sterilize rubber goods and other small items. It can be used at the end of each day, with the items wrapped and the shelves stocked and made ready for the next day. Each institution has its own physical limitations, and modifications must be made, but good nursing and medical practice should always be followed for maximum patient protection.

9
SPECIALIZED PROCEDURES

SEVERAL CATEGORIES of patients require, in addition to regular and routine care, special attention because of the nature of the surgery they have undergone. Of particular interest are thoracic, neurological, pediatric, and prostatic procedures. These will be discussed in detail.

CARE OF THE PATIENT FOLLOWING THORACOTOMY

The patient who has had an operation within his thoracic cavity has had a major interference with his normal respiratory function. Frequently, the anesthesiologist has breathed for the patient during the operative procedure to maintain his ventilation adequately. When the pleura has been opened and one, or possibly more, ribs are removed or broken, the patient needs aid in the immediate postoperative period to adjust to the changes that have been made in his pulmonary breathing apparatus. A patent airway and a clear tracheobronchial tree are vital; the patient must also have satisfactory chest cage and diaphragmatic motion. The free exchange of air into the lungs may be complicated by mucus plugs and secretions, collapse or partial collapse of lung segments, splinting of the chest because of incisional pain and collections of fluid, and blood or air in the pleural space. In addition, these patients often have an underlying disease that may or may not have been completely removed.

Several basic concepts in the care of these patients must be observed. The airway must be very closely watched and signs of respiratory distress picked up as soon as they appear. Respiratory problems may be accompanied by subcutaneous emphysema, paradoxical breathing, and deviation of the trachea from the midline. These patients are most apt to show hypoxia by restlessness, and this restlessness should be recognized as hypoxia and treated with oxygen rather than by sedation with a narcotic that will only aggravate the condition. Secretions may be a major problem and should be removed by aspiration from the pharynx, catheter aspiration from the trachea, and stir-up activity encouraging the patient to cough.

The patient should either be kept in a head-up position on his back or, when moved, turned onto the operative side. This will improve the drainage and allow freer expansion of the unoperated lung. When the patient is being turned, the drainage catheters should be checked for patency to see that they are not kinked. They can be checked by watching the excursion of the level in the tube in the drainage bottle; the tube should always be patent so that blood and air will not accumulate in the pleural space. Any accumulation will impair and impede respiratory exchange.

The blood pressure and the pulse must be watched very carefully for signs of hypovolemia, which should be treated by additional blood. Judicious use of narcotics is important to relieve incisional pain, which limits respiratory excursions and thus promotes hypoxia. Therefore, the dose of narcotics should be adjusted so that enough is given to alleviate the pain without causing respiratory depression. Postoperative x-rays should be obtained when the patient comes to the recovery room to check the expansion of the lungs. This should usually be done as soon as possible after admission and the film checked to see if any corrective measures should be taken. This will show if there is any significant residual pneumothorax or any mediastinal shift, both of which should be corrected as soon as possible. If these conditions are allowed to persist for any length of time, they will promote hypoxia, respiratory distress, and deterioration in the patient's condition. If the patient arrives in the recovery room with an endotracheal tube still in place, he should be watched carefully, preferably by the anesthetist, and tracheobronchial suction should be done as thoroughly as possible before extubation.

Treating Respiratory Distress

Signs of respiratory distress may be rapid respiration, cyanosis, and tachycardia. These signs may indicate a mucus plug in one of the major bronchi, causing a relatively massive atelectasis. Tracheal suction, encouraging the patient to cough and, in some instances, bronchoscopic removal may be required to open these air passages. The importance of rapid awakening is evident, since deep breathing and coughing will usually be sufficient to remove these secretions from the lower respiratory tract. However, if the patient cannot remove them by himself and the symptoms persist, active efforts must be made to overcome this situation. This should be done either by the anesthesiologist, the surgeon, or the bronchoscopist available for this type of work. Inhalation of Mucomyst or Alevaire has been helpful in liquidifying some of the more tenacious secretions to facilitate their expectoration. These patients should have oxygen routinely, either by nasal catheter or by mask, depending upon the individual demands. Since all of them have had major interference with their respiratory apparatus, they should be helped to maintain adequate oxygenation. If necessary, a ventilator can be used to assist respiration and to provide adequate depth and rate. However, if an assistor is used when a pneumonectomy has been done, one should remember that a lesser tidal volume should be expected and that a faster rate than normal should therefore be provided. A rate of 20 to 25 per minute should be adequate when a volume no greater than 300 to 400 cc can be achieved with part of the lung removed.

Pleural Drainage

Pleural drainage is very important and should

be watched very carefully during the immediate postoperative period. Observation of the level of fluid in the glass tube of the underwater drainage bottle and its fluctuations should show that there is a patent connection to the pleural cavity and that the patient is expanding and contracting the lung; the connection also provides a means of egress for entrapped air to eliminate any pneumothorax that may exist. It also provides a method of drainage for blood that may sometimes collect in the space following surgery. Careful attention to the amount of blood that drains through the catheter will give a basis for estimating how much should be replaced during this part of the postoperative period. Such inspection will show whether there is any massive or copious bleeding and will help determine whether this may be the cause of a deterioration of the patient's condition, the control of which might necessitate reopening of the chest. Since a patent tube performs so many functions, it is most important to determine that it is not kinked or pinched off, mechanically obstructed, or plugged by a clot. The catheter and tube should be no longer than necessary to reach from the patient's chest to the dependent drainage bottle; a long tube with many loops and ups and downs is prone to clotting, and kinking, and other forms of obstruction.

Very close cooperation among the physicians is, of course, essential for these patients; both the anesthesiologist and the surgeon should be readily available for consultation if any complications develop.

CARE OF THE PEDIATRIC PATIENT

The most common pediatric operations are tonsillectomy and adenoidectomy. On arrival in the recovery room, children subjected to these procedures should be placed in a head-down position; this can be done most conveniently by using a bolster over which the patient is draped (see Figure 8). Drainage is thereby encouraged, and there is less opportunity for the patient to collect secretions and blood in the mouth and swallow them, thus masking signs of oozing or bleeding. The patient's airway should be kept clear; the head-down position assists in maintaining the airway without artificial aids. The patient should

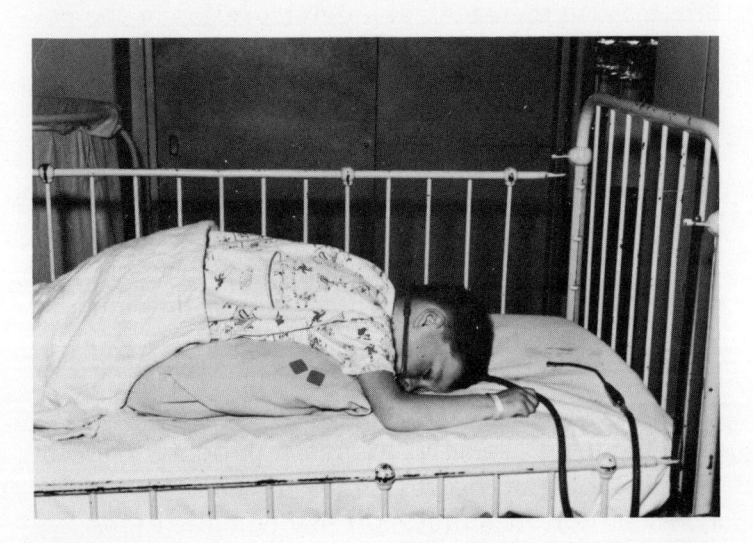

FIGURE 8
Child draped over bolster, to facilitate drainage.

be watched closely for such signs of bleeding as frequent swallowing movements and repeated expectoration of blood; increasing pulse rate, with a fall in blood pressure; air hunger; and the vomiting of large quantities of coffee-brown bloody material, showing the swallowing of blood and its dilution by gastric juices. Postoperative bleeding may either be immediate and of an amount sufficient to cause continuous expectoration, or it may be insidious as a slow ooze that may be swallowed and masked. Hemorrhaging children gradually become pale, with a rapid feeble pulse; often the first sign, other than the paleness, is the sudden vomiting of a large quantity of swallowed blood. If there is marked bleeding, the child must often be returned to the operating room and definitive measures taken to stop the bleeding. Because of the importance of watching these children in the immediate postoperative period, it is suggested that they remain in the recovery room, under the supervision of adequately trained personnel, for at least two hours following the operative procedure. During this time any bleeding will become obvious, and immediate measures can then be taken to correct the situation.

Pediatric surgery may present problems of a nature different than those encountered in adults. The air passages of children are small and may easily become obstructed. Both the airway and the character and nature of respiration should be watched very closely; shallow depth and an increase in rate are signs that trouble is brewing. Since enlarged tonsils and adenoids may cause respiratory obstruction in the anesthetized or sleeping child, special attention must be taken to assure an adequate airway, with mechanical aids if necessary.

The circulatory status of children is subject to change with the loss of relatively minor quantities of blood. Nurses who are accustomed to adults in the recovery room may not be aware that the loss of a small quantity of blood, which would be easily supported by an adult, may not be well tolerated by a child. In the immediate postoperative period, signs of pallor, tachycardia, and falling blood pressure may indicate that some blood replacement is necessary; very small amounts may often be adequate.

The temperatures of children must be very carefully watched, since hyperthermia and hyperpyrexia are not uncommon both during the operative procedure and in the immediate postoperative period. Children undergoing surgery often have an acute disease with an elevated temperature, which the drapes and operating room lights tend to increase. Therefore, the temperatures of children coming to the recovery room should be monitored as frequently as every 10 to 15 minutes until it is obvious that they will not suffer from hyperthermia. If there is any indication that the patient's temperature may rise to extraordinary levels, then hypothermia, preferably with one of the mechanical devices, should be instituted immediately to keep the patient within the range of $99°$ to $101°$ F. The patient should be carefully watched for early signs of convulsions and twitching, which frequently occur in children with markedly elevated temperatures.

Children who have undergone major surgical procedures have often been subjected to endotracheal intubation; they are much more prone than adults to laryngeal edema following the use of an endotracheal tube. Signs of stridor or edema call for steam inhalations or a croup tent. Great attention must be paid to maintaining a clear airway in the child, and any signs of laryngeal edema should be called to the attention of a physician immediately.

CARE OF THE NEUROSURGICAL PATIENT— SPECIFICALLY FOLLOWING INTRACRANIAL SURGERY

A number of important rules apply to the care of these patients. (1) Always handle the patient very gently and carefully, avoiding any rough or abrupt movements; any action that jars the patient may start intracranial bleeding or increase existing bleeding. (2) Maintain a clear airway. This is more important here than in the average case because respiratory obstruction causes hypoxia and carbon dioxide retention, which increase the venous pressure. This results in an increase in the intracranial pressure and may intensify symptoms already present or increase bleeding. (3) Patients should be discouraged from coughing and straining, since both of these increase intracranial pressure and bleeding. (4) The patient should be placed in a lateral position unless otherwise specified, since this position allows for better drainage of secretions and a better airway. (5) The patient should be watched carefully as regards his consciousness level and his orientation. The surgeon should be notified of any deterioration, increasing mental confusion, or any indication that the patient is sinking into a coma.

The doctor should be notified if there is any elevation of blood pressure associated with bradycardia; increased respiration; projectile vomiting; any fall in blood pressure with a rapid pulse and Cheyne-Stokes respiration; or any indications of neurological pathology such as weakness or paralysis, rigidity, convulsions, or fixed pupils. Extremely important are fixed and dilated pupils, since these are signs of increasing intracranial pressure and complications that may call for further surgical interference.

Since hyperpyrexia or rising temperature often indicates a neurological deterioration, the temperature should be carefully followed. The cranial orifices—the ears, nose, and mouth—should be carefully watched for any drainage of blood or spinal fluid, which may indicate the presence or location of a fracture. When the patient has reacted adequately so that there is no further danger of aspiration, the head can be elevated to improve the venous drainage and lower the intracranial pressure. Semi-Fowler's or a sitting position may be adopted if the patient is awake.

CARE OF THE ORTHOPEDIC PATIENT

Orthopedic patients very frequently come from the operating room with an extremity in a cast. The cast should leave exposed at least one finger or toe, which should be watched very carefully for the development of coldness, swelling, or cyanosis. These signs are indicative of impairment of the circulation requiring immediate correction, and the surgeon should be notified at once. The extremity should be elevated to aid venous drainage and limit swelling (see Figure 9). Undue pressure allowed to continue at a cast margin may result in injury and tissue necrosis at the pressure point. This is particularly true in the unconscious patient, who is unable to complain.

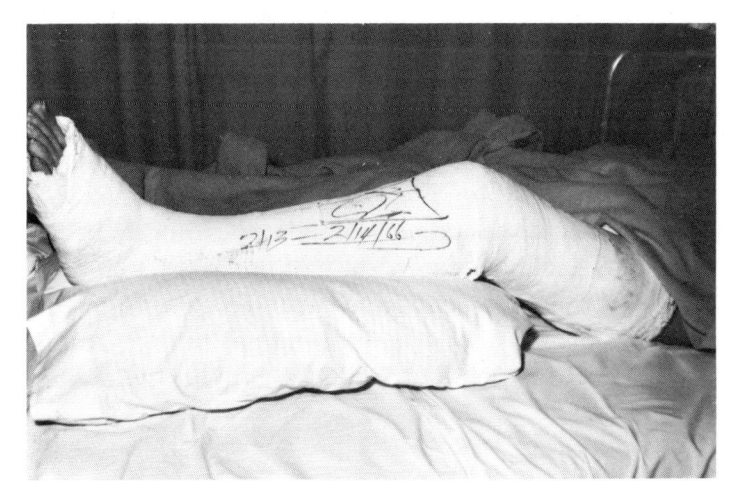

FIGURE 9
Leg with cast adequately supported with pillows.

If an open procedure has been done, the dressing or cast should be watched for bleeding. The blood pressure should be watched carefully, since hypotension and shock may occur after operations on bones, even though the blood loss was not significant. This may be caused, in some instances, by bone marrow emboli or fat emboli to the lung, resulting in respiratory embarrassment. When these patients are moved or turned, special attention should be paid to the area of the cast so that it follows naturally and does not cause any undue tension on the limb. Additional help is often required when these patients are moved, either onto their side or from the litter to the bed. If the patient is in traction, special care must be taken to see that the weights remain constant, for if they are jiggled or disturbed it will be quite painful to the patient. Any interruption to the traction should be reported immediately to the surgeon, since this may cause displacement of fracture fragments.

Patients who have had a laminectomy should be watched for bleeding; upon awakening, they should be questioned as regards neurological changes, either sensory or motor, in the extremities. If these patients are turned, the axis of the body should be kept straight and not twisted, since torsion will produce an undue strain on the operative site.

CARE OF THE UROLOGICAL PATIENT

The patients who have prostate surgery are most frequently in the older age group. On arrival in the recovery room, they have a catheter in place in the bladder for drainage. This should be watched very carefully for bleeding and the amount and character of the urine recorded. Frank blood and clots are signs of excessive bleeding. The catheter should be irrigated according to the surgeon's orders if it is not draining properly; if it becomes obstructed, the bladder becomes distended, leading to increased bleeding. Excessive bleeding should be reported and the surgeon recalled if there are any abrupt or marked changes in the patient's pulse and blood pressure.

These patients may show signs of hypertension because of hypervolemia from hemodilution. If the patient has had a transurethral prostate resection with constant irrigation of fluid, this fluid may be absorbed into the open venous sinuses and then into the bloodstream. This is followed by hemodilution and an increase in the circulating volume, which in turn causes the hypertension. This additional fluid may also overload the circulation and produce pulmonary edema and cardiac decompensation in borderline cardiac patients. The hypertension is usually followed by circulatory collapse. The hypervolemia with sodium-free irrigating fluid decreases the serum sodium to a level of mild or severe reaction. This is characterized by agitation and anxiety, restlessness, nausea, and vomiting, followed by shortness of breath, cyanosis and, in extreme cases, coma and convulsions. Treatment consists of administering hypertonic salt solutions to elevate the serum sodium while the kidneys eliminate the excess water.

10

CARDIAC ARREST

SUDDEN COLLAPSE OR ARREST

One of the most dramatic and fearsome post-anesthetic complications is cardiac arrest. It is characterized by a sudden and unexpected cessation of respiration and effective cardiac activity. The most important single factor in sudden cardiac collapse is hypoxia. This may be the result of apnea or hypoventilation due to deep anesthesia, or both; the effects of curare derivatives; or the injudicious use of narcotics. Other causes may be prone position, undetected pneumothorax, massive atelectasis, respiratory obstruction, uncontrolled coughing spasm, reflex apnea from nasoendotracheal intubation, and convulsions, particularly in hyperthermic children.

Circulatory factors that may precipitate cardiac collapse are hypotension, particularly in the older and poor-risk patient, which may lead to ventricular fibrillation and hypovolemia during the operation. Cardiac arrythmias such as paroxysmal tachycardia or heart-block may, if untreated, result in cardiac collapse. Other precipitating factors may be postoperative vomiting and aspiration causing asphyxia, acute gastric distension, and deep hypothermia, which is conducive to sudden cardiac collapse in patients who have not been adequately rewarmed before transportation to the recovery room.

DIAGNOSIS

The diagnosis of sudden collapse must be prompt and unequivocal if resuscitation is to be successful. The prophylactic use of monitors in selected cases and the frequent recording of pulse rate, blood pressure, and respiratory rate will help with quick diagnosis and give an indication of impending collapse. Warning signs are sudden disappearance of radial, carotid, or femoral pulsations; unobtainable blood pressure; pallor of skin or cyanosis; cessation of cardiac impulse; and apnea or sudden gasping respirations. When collapse is diagnosed, immediate action must follow.

Features of prophylaxis are thorough preoperative evaluation and preparation of the patient; smooth induction of anesthesia; and maintenance of anesthesia to avoid hypoxia, hypercapnia, or adverse vagal effects. Smooth emergence from anesthesia is important; excitement, respiratory obstruction, hypotension, and vomiting must be avoided or, when they occur, taken care of immediately. Lifting and positioning the patient should be done slowly, carefully, and with adequate help. Sudden jerky lifting of patients may cause precipitous hypotension or severe respiratory obstruction. The prone position must be avoided, since this may lead to respiratory obstruction not easily treated. Recovery room personnel should be briefed regarding the anesthetic, surgery performed, and specific treatments required by each patient. The anesthetist should not leave a patient in the recovery room unless he has adequate respiratory exchange.

TREATMENT

Recovery room personnel should be trained in the immediate measures to be taken when cardiac arrest occurs. The treatment of cardiac collapse involves the restoration of the two vital systems, circulation and respiration (see Figure 10). The ABC's of cardiopulmonary resuscitation are "airway, breathe, circulate." Any respiratory obstruction should be corrected, and good lung inflation must be obtained. A clear airway is vital. Maximum extension of the head is usually sufficient, but there should be no hesitancy to use an airway when necessary. Mouth-to-mouth respiration should be started immediately and continued until a bag-mask combination is obtained. Oxygen should be added to the inflating air; this alone may restore cardiac action.

Immediately upon discovery of the cardiac arrest, an emergency call must be made for help from the resuscitation team. While artificial respiration is being started, a second person must thump the precordium several times. Constant pulse monitoring should be done to check whether the heart resumes effective contraction. If no

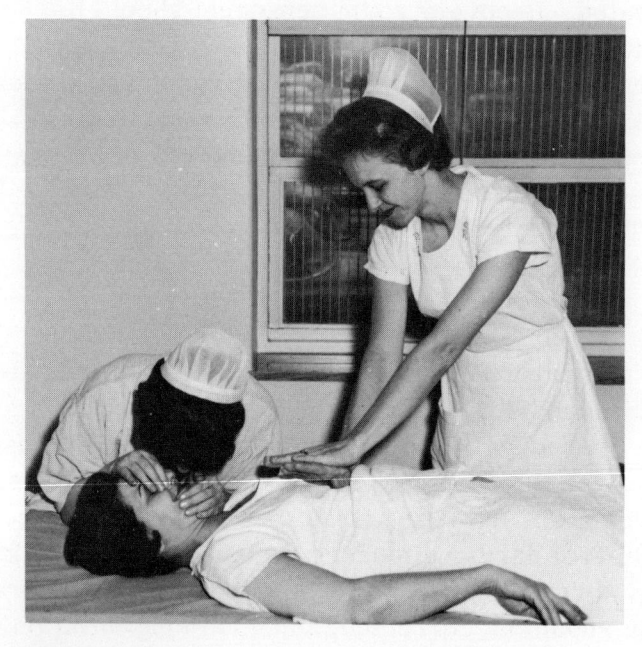

FIGURE 10
Cardiopulmonary resuscitation, with mouth-to-mouth breathing.

results are now obtained, closed cardiac massage should be started by sternal compression with the objective of achieving a rate of 60 to 80 per minute with a lung inflation at every fourth or fifth compression. If properly done, this should in most instances produce a palpable radial or femoral pulse.

As soon as a physician arrives, he should take over direction of the resuscitative efforts. If adequate circulation is not restored by closed chest massage, open thoracotomy with direct cardiac massage should be done. If ventricular fibrillation is present, a defibrillator should be used to produce cardiac standstill, followed by continued cardiac massage. Sodium bicarbonate should be given to combat the acidosis that inevitably appears with the inadequate tissue perfusion of circulatory insufficiency. Several 50-cc ampules of 3.75 gm each should be readily available. Accurate measurements of elapsed time should be made and recorded along with a timetable of the treatments as given. This is most important to judging the effects and chronology of events.

APPENDIX

LEGAL CONSIDERATIONS

The "gray area" between medical and nursing practice has been of concern to both the physician and nurse who work in a hospital recovery room. The legal right to perform medical acts must be granted through statutory law. It is not always safe for a nurse to assume that a physician's written order by itself gives her the legal right to initiate certain procedures, even in an emergency.

The American Nurses Association Committee on Nursing Practice is continuously concerned as to how they can provide assistance to nurses in problems of practice within the dependent area of nursing functions. One method of approach that has been helpful is the preparation of such joint policy statements by state nurses' associations, state medical societies, and other groups as may be appropriate for patient care procedures that fall in the "gray area" between medical and nursing practice. The American Medical Association, The American Heart Association and The American Nurses Association have encouraged this method of providing guidelines for various procedures. A statement of policy concerning patient care procedures approved by the state nursing and medical association provides a consensus of professional opinion about the proper course of action. The statement may be on any procedure that is a cause for concern to nurses within a state. It should provide criteria that can be used by hospitals and agencies within the state in setting up specific policies for their own institutions. A joint policy statement establishes a professional decision representing the considered opinions of the group involved in a patient care procedure. This is not the same as a legal decision. It does, however, provide a basis on which a legal decision may be made, should the occasion arise. Such a statement

---

*This section was prepared with the aid of Mary C. Halloran, R.N., B.S., M.S., Associate Director of Nursing, St. Luke's Hospital, New Bedford, Mass.

will not provide immunity from legal action if the nurse is negligent. However, it will give the nurse support by setting forth information which these responsible groups recognize as proper practice and procedure. All hospitals and health agencies should be encouraged to appoint committees representative of the nursing, medical, and administrative staffs to determine and implement agency policies for carrying out a procedure according to policies that have been set forth in a joint statement.

It is important for the nurse to be aware that her role in carrying out certain procedures must ultimately be determined within each state in the light of state laws and other local factors. The three main sources of information in each state to which a nurse may turn for information and assistance about her role in carrying out procedures are:

1. The state nurses association
2. The state board of registration in nursing
3. The employing agency

Joint statements have already been provided for nurses within several states.

For over twenty years the question as to whether a registered nurse may lawfully administer intravenous therapy, except in an emergency, has been a continuing concern of the nursing profession. Within the past few years, several states have solved this dilemma by issuing a joint statement covering the situation or by obtaining a ruling by the state attorney general.

Of recent concern has been the procedure for closed cardiac chest massage. Joint statements covering this procedure have been issued in this and other states. Examples of the policy statements in Massachusetts follow.

JOINT STATEMENT CONCERNING ADMINISTRATION OF INTRAVENOUS FLUIDS BY PROFESSIONAL REGISTERED NURSES*

MASSACHUSETTS NURSES ASSOCIATION
MASSACHUSETTS LEAGUE FOR NURSING

The Massachusetts Nurses Association and the Massachusetts League for Nursing in 1965 issued a "Joint Statement Concerning Administration of Intravenous Fluids by Professional Registered Nurses." The following joint statement is set forth with the objective of providing for the health and welfare of the patient and protecting the doctor, the nurse, and the employing agency. The Massachusetts Nurses Association and The Massachusetts League for Nursing believe that it is a proper part of the practice of professional registered nurses to start and administer prescribed fluids intravenously (by needle) provided that:

1. The professional registered nurse, licensed to practice nursing in Massachusetts, should have had special, competent teaching in the technique;
2. Performance of the technique should be upon the order of a licensed doctor of medicine;
3. The order should be written for a specific patient;
4. Where the technique is to be performed in a hospital or any organized agency, the procedure should be performed within the framework of designated preparation and practice of the nurse established for the hospital or agency by a committee composed of representatives from the medical staff, the department of nursing, and the administration; this framework of preparation and practice to be reproduced in writing and made available to every member of the medical and nursing staffs; and
5. It should be within the jurisdiction of that committee in a hospital or organized agency to:
    (a) decide if the nurses in the hospital or agency may perform the technique;

---

*Issued by the Massachusetts Nurses Association and the Massachusetts League for Nursing September 9, 1965.

(b) establish in-service teaching of the technique;
(c) delineate the types of fluids that nurses may administer;
(d) keep an approved list of medications that may be added to the fluid by the nurse and provide an in-service program that will acquaint the nurse with the reactions, contraindications, dosage, and results of such drugs;
(e) maintain a current list of qualified nurses on file.

JOINT STATEMENT CONCERNING THE ROLE OF THE PROFESSIONAL REGISTERED NURSE IN ADMINISTERING CLOSED CHEST CARDIOPULMONARY RESUSCITATION*

MASSACHUSETTS NURSES ASSOCIATION
MASSACHUSETTS LEAGUE FOR NURSING

The Massachusetts Nurses Association and the Massachusetts League for Nursing in 1965 issued a "Joint Statement Concerning the Role of the Professional Registered Nurse in Administering Closed Chest Cardiopulmonary Resuscitation." The following joint statement is set forth with the objective of providing for the health and welfare of the patient and protecting the doctor, the nurse, and the employing agency. The Massachusetts Nurses Association and The Massachusetts League for Nursing believe that it is a proper part of the practice of the professional registered nurse to initiate closed chest cardiopulmonary resuscitation in an emergency provided that:

1. The professional registered nurse licensed to practice in Massachusetts should have had special, competent teaching in the technique, including the recognition, understanding, and interpretation of the symptoms of cardiac arrest;
2. A physician is not immediately available to initiate the procedure;
3. A physician is notified immediately;
4. A physician, upon his arrival, should be asked to assume the responsibility for the procedure;
5. Where resuscitation, specifically respiratory and cardiac, is to be performed in a hospital or any organized agency, the procedure should be performed within the framework of designated preparation and practice of the nurse established for the hospital or agency by a committee composed of representatives from the medical staff, the department of nursing, and the administration; this framework of preparation and practice to be reproduced in writing and made available to every member of the medical and nursing staffs; and

---

*Issued by the Massachusetts Nurses Association and the Massachusetts League for Nursing September 9, 1965.

6. It should be within the jurisdiction of that committee in a hospital or organized agency to:
    (a) decide if the nurses in the hospital or agency may perform the procedure;
    (b) establish in-service teaching of the procedure and the role of the nurse;
    (c) maintain a current list of qualified nurses on file.

SUGGESTED SUPPLEMENTAL READING

Adriani, J. Techniques and Procedures of Anesthesia, 3rd edition. Springfield, Ill.: Charles C Thomas, 1964.

Adriani, J., and Parmley, J. Recovery Room. Springfield, Ill.: Charles C Thomas, 1958.

Barbour, C. M., and Little, D. M., Jr. Postoperative hypotension. J.A.M.A. 165:1529, 1957.

Bates, D. V., and Christie, R. V. Respiratory Function in Disease. Philadelphia: W. B. Saunders Co., 1964.

Beal, J. M. Manual of Recovery Room Care, 2nd edition. New York: Macmillan Co., 1962.

Bendiksen, H. H., Egbert, L. D., Hedley-Whyte, J., Laver, M. B., and Pontoppidan, H. Respiratory Care. St. Louis: C. V. Mosby, 1965.

Best, C. H., and Taylor, N. B. Physiological Basis of Medical Practice, 7th edition. Baltimore: Williams & Wilkins Co., 1961.

Comroe, J. H., Jr. The Physiology of Respiration. Chicago: Year Book Medical Publishers, 1965.

Dripps, R. D. Hazards of the immediate postoperative period. J.A.M.A. 165:795, 1957.

Goodman, L., and Gilman, A. *Pharmacological Basis of Therapeutics*, 3rd edition. New York: Macmillan Co., 1965.

Guyton, A. C. *Circulatory Physiology: Cardiac Output and Its Regulation*. Philadelphia: W. B. Saunders Co., 1963.

Hale, D. E. *Anesthesiology*, 2nd edition. Philadelphia: F. A. Davis Co., 1963.

Hamilton, W. K. Atelectasis, pneumothorax and aspiration as postoperative complications. *Anesthesiology* 22:708, 1961.

Hershey, S. G. *Shock*. Boston: Little, Brown, 1964.

Hood, R. M., and Beall, A. C., Jr. Hypoventilation, hypoxia, and acidosis occurring in the acute postoperative period. *J. Thorac. Surg.* 36:729, 1958.

Jude, J. R., and Elam, J. O. *Cardio-Pulmonary Resuscitation*. Philadelphia: F. A. Davis, 1965.

Moore, F. D. The effects of hemorrhage on body composition. *New Eng. J. Med.* 273:567, 1965.

Moore, F. D. *Metabolic Care of the Surgical Patient*. Philadelphia: W. B. Saunders Co., 1959.

Sadove, M. S., and Cross, J. H. *Recovery Room*. Philadelphia: W. B. Saunders Co., 1956.

Stephenson, H. E. *Cardiac Arrest and Resuscitation*, 2nd edition. St. Louis: C. V. Mosby Co., 1964.

INDEX

Abdominal operations, and after-effects of spinal anesthesia, 82
Acidosis
 in cardiac arrest, treatment, 113
 respiratory, 53, 91
 in shock, treatment, 73-74
Adenoidectomy, 100-103
Admission, procedure for, 13-14, 85-86
Airway, 29-30
 insertion of, 48, 49
 obstruction, 51-52
 removal of, 50-51
 role of, 50-51
Alevaire, 98
Allergic patient, 54
Allergic reaction to blood transfusion, 88, 89
 treatment, 89
Alpha-blocking agents, 73
Alveolar wall, 39
Alveoli, 38
 pulmonary edema in, 44
Ambu bag, 53, 78
American Heart Association, 115
American Medical Association, 115
American Nurses Association, 115
American Nurses Association Committee on Nursing Practice, 115
Aminophyllin, 54
Amyl nitrite, 91
Anemic anoxia, 45, 46-47
 treatment, 46-47
Anesthesia
 classification, 75
 effects of, 64-65
 general, 75
 inhalation, 75-79
 intravenous, 75, 79-80
 narcotic, 75, 79
 rectal, 75, 80-81
 spinal, 75, 81-82
Anesthesia department, 3, 5
Anesthesia record, 13
Anesthesiologist in the recovery room, 12
 role of, 5-6
Anesthetist, nurse, 10-11
Anoxia
 anemic, 45, 46-47
 anoxic, 43-45, 47
 from complete laryngospasm, 37
 histotoxic, 46-47
 stagnant, 45-46, 47
Anoxic anoxia, 43-45
 treatment, 47
Anxiety
 sign of decreased serum sodium reaction, 107
 sign of hypoxemia, 52
 sign of shock, 67, 69, 74
Apnea
 and carbon dioxide decrease, 42
 and cardiac arrest, 109, 110
Aramine, 73
Arfonad, 91
Arterial elasticity, 61, 62

Arterial pressure. See Blood pressure
Asphyxia, resultant, 48, 109
Aspiration, 52
　causing asphyxia, 109
　fluid, 51
　of foreign bodies, 37
　late complications of, 51
Asthma, 38
Asthmatic attack, and respiratory obstruction, 44
Asthmatic patient, 54
Atelectasis, 52
　following aspiration, 51
　massive, and cardiac arrest, 109
　prevention through deep breathing, 56, 86
　prevention following rectal anesthesia, 80
Avertin, 75

Barbiturates, intravenous, 79-80
　recovery from, 80
Beds, disadvantages of, 23-24
Bladder drainage, following prostate surgery, 107
Blankets, 25
Bleeding, excessive, following prostate surgery, 107
Blood
　frank, 107
　frozen stored, 72
　oozing, 90
　in the urine, 90
Blood expanders, 72
Blood flow, resistance to, 62
Blood loss
　and cardiovascular depressants, 64
　during operative procedure, 45, 64
　following general anesthetics, 43
　following tonsillectomy or adenoidectomy, 102
　and hypotension, 63, 91
Blood pressure, 60-63
　control of, 62
　cuffs and manometers, 31
　during respiratory obstruction, 50
　following neurosurgery, 104
　following orthopedic surgery, 106
　following thoracotomy, 97
　measurement, 60-61
　purposes, 59
　unobtainable, and cardiac arrest, 110
Blood replacement, following thoracotomy, 99
Blood stagnation, 46
Blood transfusion reactions, 88-90
　allergic, 88, 89
　febrile, 88, 89
　hemolytic, 88, 89
　producing a shock-like state, 91
　treatment, 90
Blood vessels, 60-63
Blood viscosity, 62
Blood volume, 62, 63
　measurement, in shock, 70
　reduction in, 64, 91, 97
Bradycardia in the neurosurgical patient, 104
Breathing
　deep, 56, 57, 86
　obstructed, 90. See also Respiratory obstruction
　paradoxical, 48, 96
　See also Respiration
Brevital, 75
Bronchi, 38
Bronchial tree, 38
Bronchiectasis, 53
Bronchioles, 38
Bronchitis, 53
Bronchoconstriction, 52-56
　diagnosis of, 54
　due to fluid aspiration, 51
　treatment, 54
Bronchospasm, 51
　cause of respiratory obstruction, 44
　treatment, 54

Carbon dioxide
  elimination, 55-56, 64-65
  flow through alveolar wall, 39
  levels, effect on respiration, 42
Cardiac accelerator nerves, 62
Cardiac arrest
  causes of, 109
  diagnosis, 110-111
  immediate measures, 111
  measurements, 113
  prophylaxis, 110
  treatment, 111-113
  warning signs, 110
Cardiac-arrest tray, 30
Cardiac arrythmias, 109
Cardiac decompensation, 107
Cardiac impulse, cessation of, and cardiac arrest, 110
Cardiac massage, 112-113
Cardiac output, 62
Cardiac patients, 107
Cardiopulmonary resuscitation, 111-112
  joint statement concerning, 116, 119-120
Cardiovascular depressants, 64
Cast, 106
  margin, pressure at, 105
Caudal anesthesia, 75
Central venous pressure, measurement in shock, 70
Cerebral dysfunction in shock, 69
Charge for patient service, basis of, 14-15
Charting desk, 19
Charts, 26-27
Chest constriction, 38
Cheyne-Stokes respiration, 104
Children. See Pediatric patient
Chill, following blood transfusion, 89
Chlorpromazine, 73
Circulation, 5
  anatomy, 59-63
  failing, in stagnant anoxia, 45-46
  physiology, 59-63

Circulation impairment, in orthopedic patient, 105
  treatment, 105
Circulatory system, 59
Clots, 107
Coma, due to decreased serum sodium, 107
Consciousness level, following neurosurgery, 104
Convulsions
  and cardiac arrest, 109
  due to decreased serum sodium, 107
  following neurosurgery, 104
  in the pediatric patient, 102-103
Cortisone, in shock therapy, 74
Cough stimulation, 56, 57, 86
Coughing spasm, uncontrolled, and cardiac arrest, 109
Croup tent, 103
Curare derivatives, and cardiac arrest, 109
Curarization, cause of respiratory depression, 55
Curarized patients, care of, 54-55
Cyanosis
  and cardiac arrest, 110
  due to decreased serum sodium, 107
  resulting from complete laryngospasm, 37
  resulting from respiratory obstruction, 50
Cyclopropane, 65, 75
  recovery from, 76-77
Cyclopropane shock, 65, 77

Death, imminent, 13
Deep breathing, 56, 57, 86
Delirium
  emergence, 76, 91
  treatment, 76
  following cyclopropane anesthesia, 76
  treatment, 76
Demerol, 75
Diastolic pressure, 61

Dibenzyline, 73
Discharging the patient, 14
Diuresis, following spinal
 anesthesia, 82
Doxapram hydrochloride, 32,
 55
Drainage
 following neurosurgery, 104
 following thoracotomy, 96
 pleural, 98-99
Dressings, 33
 on orthopedic patient, 106
Drug supply, 31-32
Dyspnea, 38

Edema
 cause of respiratory
  obstruction, 44
 following blood transfusion,
  89
  treatment, 89
 laryngeal, 103
  treatment, 103
 pulmonary, 44, 107
Electric muscle stimulator, 55
Electrocardiogram, 60
Electronic equipment, 33-34
Emergence delirium, 76, 91
 treatment of, 76
Emphysema, 53, 96
Endotracheal tray, 29
Endotracheal tube, removal of,
 50-51
Ether, 75
 recovery from, 77
Ethyl chloride, 75, 78
Exercising the patient, 56-57
Expiration, 39, 40, 42

Febrile reaction to blood
 transfusion, 88, 89
Fibrosis, 53
Financial considerations, 14-15
Fluid absorption syndrome, 90
Fluid administration, sets for,
 29-31
Fluid aspiration, 51
Fluid irrigation, with trans-
 urethral prostate
 resection, 107

Fluothane, 75
 recovery from, 77-78
Fowler's position, 31, 104
Frank blood, 107

Gallamine, 83
Gas sterilizer, 93
Gasping respirations, and
 cardiac arrest, 110
Gastric contents, inhalation
 of, 44
General anesthetics, 75
 and respiratory depression,
  43

Halloran, Mary C., 115n.
Halothane, recovery from,
 77-78
Hand-squeezing test, 54, 83
Head extension, treatment for
 respiratory obstruction,
 48
Head-lifting test, 54, 83
Heart failure, 46, 63
Heart function, 59-60
Heart rate, 60
 regulation of, 62
Heart-block, 109
Hematocrit determination, 70
Hemodilution following
 prostate surgery, 107
Hemolytic reaction to blood
 transfusion, 89
Hemorrhage, 68
 in the pediatric patient, 101
Hemothorax, 41
Hering-Breuer reflex, 42
Histotoxic anoxia, 46
 treatment, 47
Humidification of inspired
 air, 36
Hydrocortisone, 54
Hypercapnia, 55
Hypercarbia, under cyclo-
 propane anesthesia, 76
Hyperpyrexia
 following neurosurgery, 104
 in the pediatric patient, 102
Hypertension, postoperative,
 90-91

Index / 127

causes of, 90-91
following prostate surgery, 107
treatment, 91
Hyperthermia, in the pediatric patient, 102-103
Hypertonic salt solutions, 107
Hypervolemia, following prostate surgery, 107
Hypotension, postoperative, 65, 91-92
  a blood transfusion reaction, 90
  from disturbance in blood volume, 63
  following cyclopropane anesthesia, 76
  in the older patient, 109
  and postural changes, 91
  treatment and immediate measures, 92
Hypothermia, and cardiac arrest, 109
Hypoventilation, 51-57
  cause of blood pressure rise, 90
  diagnostic aids in, 55
  following use of muscle relaxants, 83
  treatment of, 78
Hypovolemia, 64, 91, 97
Hypoxemia
  early signs of, 52
  treatment, 52, 66
Hypoxia, 52-56, 66
  and cardiac arrest, 109
  caused by pain, 53-54, 66
  following use of muscle relaxants, 45
  following thoracotomy, 41, 96
  in old-aged patients, 53
  and respiratory obstruction, 47
  and respiratory stimulation, 42

Infection prevention and control, 92-93
Inhalation anesthesia, 75-79

Inhalation therapy department, 32-33
Inspiration, 39, 40, 42
Intensive care unit, 1
Intercostal muscles, paralysis of, 82, 83
Intracranial pressure
  rise, 90
  signs of, following neurosurgery, 103-104
Intracranial surgery, 103. See also Neurosurgical patient
Intravenous anesthesia, 75, 79-80
Intravenous extension set, 70
Intravenous perfusion, 75
  reaction from and treatment, 82
Intravenous therapy procedure, joint statement concerning, 116, 117-118
Isuprel, 54

Jaw elevation, treatment for respiratory obstruction, 48

Lactated Ringer's solution, in treatment of shock, 73
Laminectomy, 106
Laryngeal edema, 103
  treatment, 103
Laryngopharynx, 36
Laryngospasm, 37
  cause of respiratory obstruction, 44
  following barbiturates, 80
Larynx, 37
Legal considerations, 115-116
Levophed, 73
Linens, 33
Litters, advantages of, 23

Massachusetts League for Nursing, 117, 119
Massachusetts Nurses Association, 117, 119
Mediastinal shift, 97
Minute volume, of oxygen, 41

Monitors
  minimum required unit, 33
  use of, 110
Mouth breathing, 36
Mouth-to-mouth respiration, 111, 112
Moving the patient, 56-57, 86-87
Mucomyst, 98
Muscle relaxants, 75, 83
  cause of respiratory obstruction, 45
  effects of, 43
Muscular tonus, evaluation of, 54
Music, in the recovery room, 28

Narcotic anesthesia, 75, 79
Narcotics
  administration of, 91
  and cardiac arrest, 109
  complications following, 87
  for shock patients, 74
Nasal mucosa, 35-36
Nasopharynx, 36
Nausea, postoperative, 76
  due to decreased serum sodium, 107
Neo-Synephrine, 73
Nerve blocks, 75
Neurogenic disturbances, 68
Neurosurgical patient
  blood pressure, 104
  bradycardia in, 104
  care of, 103-104
  consciousness level, 104
  convulsions, 104
  drainage in, 104
  fixed and dilated pupils, 104
  fracture indicated, 104
  handling, 103
  hyperpyrexia in, 104
  intracranial pressure in, 103-104
  paralysis, 104
  positioning, 104
  pulse, 104
  respiration, 104
  respiratory obstruction in, 103
  rigidity, 104
  temperature, 104
  weakness, 104
Nisentil, 75, 79
Nitrous oxide, 75
  recovery from, 78-79
Norepinephrine, 62
Nose, 35-36
Nurse
  anesthetist, 10-11
  graduate, 11
  head. See Supervisor
  operating room, 12
  private duty, 12-13
  role of, 6-7
  student, 8
Nurse's aides, 11
Nurse's station, 19, 26-27
Nursing procedures
  information sources for, 116
  legal considerations, 115-116

Obstructed breathing, 90. See also Respiratory obstruction
Oliguria, 69
Operating room nurses, training in the recovery room, 12
Operating room supervisor, 3, 7
Orders, postoperative, 13-14
Oropharyngeal airway. See Airway
Oropharyngeal muscle tone, 36
Oropharyngeal tract, occlusion of, 47-48
Oropharynx, 36
Orthopedic patient
  blood pressure, 106
  care of, 105-106
  circulation impairment in, 105
    treatment, 105
  dressing, 106
  handling, 106
Oxygen, flow through the alveolar wall, 39
Oxygen administration
  facilities, 22-23, 25-26
  following thoracotomy, 98

Index / 129

for hypotension, 92
for shock, 74
Oxygen levels, effect on
    respiration, 42
Oxygen supply, minute volume
    of, 41
Oxygen withdrawal, 92

Paralysis following neuro-
    surgery, 104
Paroxysmal tachycardia, 109
Patient
    admission to recovery room,
        13-14, 85-86
    allergic, 54
    anxiety. See Anxiety
    asthmatic, 54
    contamination, 92-93
    discharge of, 14
    exercising, 56-57
    in extremis, 13
    handling, 65-66, 110
        following neurosurgery,
            103
        following orthopedic
            surgery, 106
        following spinal anesthesia,
            81
    initial care of, 65-66
    mobilization, 56, 57, 65-66,
        86-87
    neurosurgical. See Neuro-
        surgical patient
    position changes, 56-57, 86
    positioning of, 31
        following neurosurgery,
            104
        following spinal anesthesia,
            81
        following thoracotomy, 96
        following tonsillectomy or
            adenoidectomy, 100
    restlessness. See Restless-
        ness
Patients, arrangement of,
    18-19, 22-24
Pediatric patient
    blood loss, signs of, 102
    care of, 100-103
    convulsions, 102-103
        and cardiac arrest, 109

hemorrhaging, 101
and laryngeal edema, 103
    treatment, 103
positioning of, 100
respiratory distress,
    101-102
segregation of, 19, 22
temperature control, 102
Penthrane, 75
    recovery from, 77-78
Personnel health, 92
Personnel policies, 9-10
Personnel schedule, 9-10
Personnel training, 3-4
Petechiae, 90
Pharyngeal suction, 26
Pharynx, 36-37
Pheochromocytoma, 91
Physician, role of, 13-14
Pleural cavity, 40-41
Pleural drainage
    after thoracotomy, 98
    patent tube, 99
Pneumonectomy, respiratory
    assistance rate, 98
Pneumonia, resultant, 51
Pneumonitis, resultant, 51
Pneumothorax, 41, 97, 99, 109
Position, prone, 110
Position changes, patient,
    56-57, 86
Positioning the patient. See
    Patient, positioning of
Postoperative orders, 13-14
Postsurgical room, 1
Postural changes, and hypo-
    tension, 91
Preoperative medication, 64
Preoperative narcotics, and
    respiratory depression,
    43, 44-45
Private duty nurses, 12-13
Prone position, and cardiac
    arrest, 109, 110
Prostate surgery, 106-107
Pulmonary edema, 44, 107
Pulmonary emboli, 92
Pulmonary ventilation, index
    of, 41
Pulse
    arrhythmic, 90

Pulse—Continued
 disappearance of, and cardiac arrest, 110
 following thoracotomy, 97
 monitoring, in cardiac arrest, 111
 pressure, 61
  following neurosurgery, 104
 rate
  rapid, 64, 104
  in shock, 70
  slow, 50
  slow bounding, 91
Pupils, fixed and dilated, following neurosurgery, 104

Recovery room
 admission to, 13-14, 85-86
 architectural layout of, 21
 arrangement, 18-19, 24
 chart, 27
 costs, 14-15
 death in, 13
 defined, 1-2
 discharge from, 14
 heat regulation, 24-25
 location, 3, 7, 17-18
 management, 10-13
 need for, 2-3
 part of the operating room, 3, 6-7
 personnel, 3-4, 9-10, 92
 physical arrangements, 22-24
 a postanesthesia room, 1-2
 schedule, 9-10
 supervision of, 5, 6-7
 supervisor, 7-8, 12, 13-14
Rectal anesthesia, 75, 80-81
Regional anesthesia, 75, 81-82
Regitine, 91
Resident, training in the recovery room, 12
Respiration, 5
 anatomy of, 35-38
 chemical factors in control of, 42
 in curarized patients, 54-55
 during the operation, 56
 external, 35
 following neurosurgery, 104
 following spinal anesthesia, 82
 gasping, and cardiac arrest, 110
 and humidification, 36
 internal, 35
 inverse, 48, 96
 manual control, 32
 mechanically assisted, 53
 mechanics of, 39-41
 mouth-to-mouth, 111, 112
 noisy, 47, 48
 normal, 48, 50
 organs of, 35-38
 rate of, 41
  following pneumonectomy, 98
 regulation of, 41-42
 rhythmicity of, 42
 under anesthesia, 56
 and ventilation, 51-57
Respirators, 32
Respiratory acidosis, 53, 91
Respiratory assistance, 78
 following pneumonectomy, 98
 following rectal anesthesia, 80
 following thoracotomy, 95
 following use of muscle relaxants, 83
Respiratory center, 41-42
Respiratory depression
 caused by curarization, 55
 caused by preoperative narcotics, 43, 44-45
 and general anesthetics, 43
Respiratory distress
 following thoracotomy, 95-98
 signs of, 97
 treatment, 97-98
 following tonsillectomy or adenoidectomy, 101-102
 See also Respiratory obstruction
Respiratory exchange, limited, and obese patients, 54

Respiratory obstruction, 36-37, 47-51, 90
 and blood pressure, 50
 and cardiac arrest, 109
 causes of, 43-45
 checking for, 50
 following barbiturates, 80
 following edema reaction, 89
 following neurosurgery, 103
 and secretions, 51
 tongue in, 47-48
 treatment of, 48-49
 See also Respiratory distress
Respiratory problems, 51-52
Respiratory stimulant, 55
Restlessness
 due to decreased serum sodium, 107
 following thoracotomy, 96
 sign of blood transfusion reaction, 90
 sign of hypoxemia, 52
Resuscitators, 32
Rigidity, following neurosurgery, 104

Secretions
 removal from lower respiratory tract, 97-98
 and respiratory obstruction, 51
Sedatives, complications following, 87
Serum sodium reaction, 107
 treatment, 107
Shock, 66-74
 during anesthesia, 64, 65
 blood pressure in, 69
 blood replacement in, 72
 blood volume measurement, 70
 bodily compensation for, 67
 causes of, 67-68
 cerebral dysfunction in, 69
 compensated, 71
 defined, 66
 diagnosis of, 68-70
 management of, 70-74
 oliguria in, 69

 prevention of, 71
 signs of, 66-67
 skin condition in, 69
 tests for, 70
 thirst in, 69
 treatment, 72-74
Shortness of breath, due to decreased serum sodium, 107
Skin, flushed, 89
Skin condition in shock, 69
Skin pallor, and cardiac arrest, 110
Skin rash, 89
Snoring, 47, 48
Sodium Pentothal, 79-80
 recovery from, 80
Sodium thiopental, 75
Sphygmomanometer, 61
Spinal anesthesia, 75, 81-82
 effect of, 43
 after abdominal operations, 82
 injection of, 81
 recovery from, 81-82
Stagnant anoxia, 45-46, 47
Steam inhalation, 103
Sterilization, 93
Sternal compression, 112
"Stir-up" regime, 56, 86-88
 following Fluothane anesthesia, 78
Stretchers, advantages of, 23
Student nurses, in the recovery room, 8
Succinylcholine, 83
Suctioning, 56, 86, 87-88
 facilities, 22-23, 25-26
 following rectal anesthesia, 81
Supervisor, role of, 7-8, 12, 13-14
Surgical shock, hypotension in, 91
Surital, 75
Swallowing
 effect on larynx, 37
 effect on pharynx, 36
Systolic pressure, 61

Tachycardia, 64, 90
  paroxysmal, 109
  in shock, 66, 67, 69, 70
Temperature, following
    neurosurgery, 104
Temperature control, 24-25
  following tonsillectomy or
    adenoidectomy, 102
Thirst, in shock, 69
Thoracic cage
  enlargement of, 40
  restricted movement of,
    54
Thoracotomy
  care following, 95-99
  and pleural drainage,
    98-99
  and respiratory distress,
    95-98
  treatment, 97-98
Thoracotomy set, 29-30
Thyroid crisis, 91
Tidal air, rate of, 41
Tissue perfusion, in shock
    therapy, 73
Tissue trauma, 68
Tongue
  and respiratory obstruction, 47-48
  rolling back, 36
Tonsillectomy, 22, 26,
    100-103
Trachea, 38
  deviation of, 96
Tracheostomy, and artificial
    humidification, 36
Tracheotomy set, 29-30
Traction, interruption to, 106

Transurethral prostate resection and hemodilution,
    107
Trendelenburg position, 31
  for hypotension, 92
Tubocurarine, 83

Urological patient, care of,
    106-107
Utility room, 29

Vagus nerves, 62
Vascular bed, 62, 63
Vasomotor nerves, 62
Vasopressor drugs, 32
  use in shock treatment, 73
Ventilation, 51-57
Ventricular fibrillation, in
    cardiac arrest, 113
Vinethene, 75
Visitors, 13
Vocal cords
  closed, 44
  contraction of, 37
  stimulation of, 80
Volatile inhalation anesthetics,
    75
Vomiting, 76
  and cardiac arrest, 109
  due to decreased serum
    sodium, 107
  projectile, 104
Vomitus, cause of respiratory
    obstruction, 44

Weakness, following neurosurgery, 104
Wheezing, 54